Resilient

Hope For Healing
From My Journey
To Yours

Susan Ledet, PT, ND

WESTBOW
PRESS®
A DIVISION OF THOMAS NELSON
& ZONDERVAN

WestBow Press books may be ordered through booksellers or by contacting:

WestBow Press
A Division of Thomas Nelson & Zondervan
1663 Liberty Drive
Bloomington, IN 47403
www.westbowpress.com
1 (866) 928-1240

ISBN: 978-1-5127-2596-4 (sc)
ISBN: 978-1-5127-2597-1 (e)

Library of Congress Control Number: 2015921450

Print information available on the last page.

WestBow Press rev. date: 1/7/2016

CONTENTS

About The Author vii

Introduction ix

Chapter 1   My Awareness Begins 1

Chapter 2   A Near Death Experience 7

Chapter 3   Spiritual Healing 11

Chapter 4   Emotional Blocks and How They are
             Connected to Physical Pain 14

Chapter 5   More Answers and A Revelation 16

Chapter 6   Healing According to My Will 23

Chapter 7   Healing According to the Will of God 25

Chapter 8   A Turning Point 30

Chapter 9   A Renewed Strength 32

Chapter 10   Spiritual Healing 36

Chapter 11   Emotional Healing 38

Chapter 12   Generational Curses 44

Chapter 13   Guidance Through The Holy Spirit 46

Chapter 14   Identity Crisis 59

Chapter 15   Re-Patterning My Nervous System 65

Chapter 16   The Core of My Healing 72

Chapter 17   Shocking Answers!! 74

Chapter 18   Rejection All Over Again 79

Chapter 19   Marriage Encounter Weekend 84

Chapter 20   Apls- Another Answer 87

Chapter 21 Back to My Passion.. 100
Chapter 22 A Mystery Revealed 103
Chapter 23 Logic or Truth.. 108

Acknowledgements 115
Bibliography...119

ABOUT THE AUTHOR

I was born the youngest of 8 in the beautiful state of Maine and at age 9 moved to Oklahoma with my family due to my father's work. I married my high school sweetheart (even though we were from rival schools) at age 22. We have been married 20 years and have 7 children. I graduated from McLoud High School in 1988 and earned a Bachelors degree of Medical Biology from Southeastern Oklahoma State by May of 1992. I continued my studies at the Oklahoma Health Science Center and earned my Bachelors degree in Physical Therapy in 1995. I have managed my private practice, Quality Physical Therapy since 2000, with a specialty in manual therapy techniques treating patients as a whole: body, mind, and spirit. We have homeschooled our children for the past 5 years and plan to continue until the last has graduated.

I have lived with chronic pain. Some of my injuries and ailments include but are not limited to: premature birth with a hyaline membrane with a minimal chance of survival, many sprained ankles, a broken ankle, jammed fingers, chronic headaches, TMJ dysfunction, urinary track infections, chronic nausea, dizziness, fainting episodes, fractures of the lumbar spine, disc herniations of the lumbar and thoracic spine, congenital hip dysplasia (a partially dislocated hip at birth) not found until age 36, biceps tendonitis, rotator cuff tear, detached labrum of the hip, wrist sprain, hormone imbalance, end-stage adrenal fatigue, neural cardiogenic syncope (a nerve causing abnormal heart rate and faint episodes for unknown reason), tachycardia (rapid heart rate), and low blood pressure. Otherwise normal and healthy!!!! I may have left some out, but you get the point, I am not a hypochondriac. I believe these injuries and ailments are generational (physical, emotional, and spiritual). As my father once said jokingly "you got what was left" Little did he know he was speaking much truth. God has blessed me with these ailments and given me the strength and courage to learn from them and share my knowledge with others so they may be inspired in their healing journey. My passion in life is being a wife, mother, and healer.

It was my own healing journey that led me to continue my studies in 2008-2009, earning my certificate of Nutritional Counseling and Doctorate of Naturopathy. Through much work and the grace of God, Quality Physical Therapy became Quality Physical Therapy and Wellness in 2010.

INTRODUCTION

Do you ever wonder why some people never get sick with a cold or the flu yet they end up with cancer? Or how an innocent child by the age of 2 can have Leukemia? And how did Grandpa Joe grow up on steak and potatoes and remain healthy as an ox, while his sons and daughters were ill with liver and kidney disease by their early 40's? How does a healthy mother of 8 not so healthy children have granddaughters who can not reproduce? Why is a child created perfectly in God's image born with jaundice? Could it be related to mom and dad's diet? Where does mental illness come from? What is the real source of anxiety, depression, schizophrenia and bipolar disorder? Do you ever wonder why you have no sex drive? Sure, maybe your hormones are out of balance, but why? Could these have been inherited genetically? Are there emotional blocks that keep your brain from stimulating the endocrine system from releasing hormones? Have you done something to offend God? Maybe it's all the above. I believe there are answers to all these questions.

There are many things that influence our health physically, emotionally and spiritually. Life begins at conception, and at that same moment, the genes that are passed to the child are affected by the food our mothers and fathers consume, toxins of the environment, old family secrets, emotional blocks, spiritual battles, etc. These influences can be passed through several generations. Our patterning in life begins at this first moment, as we are carried in our mother's womb. It is here that we begin our journey and form our life habits; so it does make a difference to us if we started out as a planned or an unwanted pregnancy. Generational curses started with the original sin of Adam and Eve; however, we can choose to continue to sin and decrease quality of our health, or change the way we live and work toward the kingdom of God, thus preventing illness and reversing disease not only our present generation but generations past and generations of the future. God does not intend for us to live with fear, pain, depression, anxiety or any illness that keeps us from Him. He says in Hebrews 13:15 *"I will never forsake or abandon you"*.

I would like to share my knowledge, as well as my journey of healing, and how it has affected my physically, emotionally, and spiritually health. I have truly felt inspired to share this with you. I am so grateful to be able on this journey, so that I may be a servant of God, and through Him, to continue to heal and bring knowledge to all those who read this or cross my path. I pray this book will help many find peace and resources they need for their healing. Healing others through God's work is a passion of mine. To keep this healing and knowledge to myself would be a sin. It is said in Hosea 4:6 *"My people perish for want of knowledge! Since you have rejected knowledge, I will reject you from my priesthood; since you have ignored the law of your God, I will also ignore your sons."*

I encourage all who have knowledge to share it, so that we may carry out the will of God. After all, we are on this earth for only a short while. Our purpose before leaving to live with Him forever, is to bring Him glory by carrying out His will for our lives. I prayed for so long to have answers for my patients and my family, to know why they suffered from similar ailments, and to find the answers to their healing. I wanted to "fix" everyone. God gave me and continues to give me opportunities to gain knowledge and find answers through my own healing journey. I have openly shared some of my journal entries throughout this book.

CHAPTER 1

My Awareness Begins

JOURNAL ENTRY: 3-18-07 *I feel the need to journal, yet I don't know where to begin. Well, I guess I will just start with the present and see where it takes me. I can't seem to stop the tears since yesterday. They are still rolling as I write, but deep inside it feels good to get them out, even though I am feeling very sad. I know now after 10 long years of chronic pain how I have survived... not only survived but feel blessed by the pain... I have endured and still endure. I thank God for his strength, for his love, for never abandoning me. He has shown me, and continues to show me, great things through my pain, and I feel his presence closer each day. The stiles-mines course this weekend has opened up a very deep part of my pain that I have waited a long time for. I feel I am finally reaching that final chapter in my life that will free me from this chronic pain and help me to be whole and a great healer through God's hands. Through all my years of pain, I think I am finally experiencing core pain that Micha taught me a long*

> *time ago when she first started treating me (sometime in 1998). I thank God for Micha always giving me that piece of hope just when I needed it. I never dreamed my pain could be worse than it had been in the past several years with my back. The pain in my arm these past two or three weeks just about broke me. It has been so intense I don't know how I kept functioning, much less treating other patients, cooking, and caring for my family. God gave me the strength to keep going, but I know now I have to take time to heal myself so that I can be a better healer, be whole again, be the wife, mother, friend and therapist God wants me to be. I pray I can let go soon and have the grace to ask for the help I need, and to let go of whatever is holding me back so I can be free. As I write, my pain in my shoulder and wrist is increasing so I better take a break and try more prayer for now. I need support, but don't know how or where to get it yet.*

The core of our healing almost always has an emotional and spiritual component. Manual Physical Therapists often describe healing as "peeling the layers of an onion", saying, "the closer you get to the core the more it makes you cry". Emotionally, I have held in the feelings I had. This was a pattern of behavior I had as a small child, which had been inherited by many generations before my own. The saying, "You live what you learn" holds a lot of truth. The patterning we develop in-utero is received for a reason, just as the strength and courage that God gives us throughout our life. This patterning forms who we become, good or bad. The important part is what we do with that patterning we received early in life. We can grow from it and gain knowledge, carrying out God's will for us, or we can dwell on the 'bad genes' or 'rough life' we grew up with. All the tools we need for a life of peace are within us; we can use them or let them rust.

JOURNAL ENTRY 3-19-07 *I keep trying, but I can't focus on anything. My mind is racing. I have had so many thoughts going through my head, are they real? I'm not sure yet. I think I know why Sammy (my 6 month old son at the time) is not sleeping. We share the same pain. I pray I can find the answers so we can be healed. It seems crazy but it makes sense. I thank Margo for praying with me today. It has helped. I pray I sleep tonight; I really need to sleep for my healing. I am scared of what I hold inside, but excited to release it so I can go on and this pain will leave me. I feel part of me is dying inside, and it hurts so badly.*

During this time in my healing, I began to realize a lot of my symptoms were signs of what is called 'sympathetic shock', which means an experience that overwhelms our body/mind system, as defined by Dr. Stephanie Mines, Ph.D. I first met Dr. Mines at a course I chose to attend as part of my continuing education. She teaches healing techniques utilizing energy medicine through what is called the TARA Approach or Jin Shin Tara. At this time I was about 3 months pregnant with my fifth child. He was totally unexpected, but worth every minute. Before I found out I was pregnant, my four-year old son Lucas told me I was pregnant, and I laughed and told him, "No, I'm not". Well, two weeks later, I found out I was. This pregnancy was different, I felt the baby move very early, (about 10 weeks) and I had the feeling I was carrying twins, it was a very strong feeling. About 2 months into the pregnancy, my son Lucas told me "there are two babies in your tummy and they are boys" I was speechless. He was very insistent, and when I went for an ultrasound the doctor said there was only one baby and Lucas argued "No, there are two boys". I did not disregard what he was saying, because it actually confirmed what I was feeling. I decided we would wait, because a twin is sometimes missed on an ultrasound that early. Well, at about 3 months along, while I was in the course, I went to the bathroom, and I noticed a white piece of tissue-looking substance I passed after going to the bathroom. At that point I had a funny sensation and was hesitant to flush the toilet. But I did, and I tried to forget about it. Later that week, I asked Lucas if there were still 2 boys in my tummy. He bluntly declared, "No. One boy died". Again, I was speechless. How could a four-year old come up with something like this? I spent the rest of the pregnancy quietly denying that I had lost a twin, but I continued to have a sense of loss.

As I completed the course and received the treatments, layers of emotional pain began surfacing. For example, the pain in my shoulder revealed some held-in emotions I had from losing my brother earlier in my life. As the therapist worked on my shoulder, tears began to fall uncontrollably and memories of my brother began to surface. I never took the time to grieve when he passed away. He died at the age of 33 from a cancerous brain tumor. At that time, I was 22, preparing for my wedding, and getting ready to begin Physical Therapy School. He died just a month before my wedding, so there were many mixed emotions during that season. I never realized how much anger and hurt I had held in until it surfaced during these treatments, 14 years later. When I started crying, I thought I would never stop. More emotions surfaced during another physical therapy session with Micha and Margo and another layer of my shoulder pain was removed. This would be the beginning of many layers.

> JOURNAL ENTRY: 3-20-07 *I finally feel safe and have the ability to move on. I know it is not over, but I now know I did have a piece of me dying inside - I lost Sammy's twin brother (given the name Michael, in my awareness) several months ago. Through God's strength, I was able to let him go home today. He is with his Uncle Ray (my brother I lost to cancer) now, and I know we will all be together again one day. Now I can*

*finally face the truth that has been burning within me. I
pray God will keep us all close and help us through this
difficult time. I know he is always by my side. I finally
had the courage to talk to Doug about Michael. I am so
thankful he is my husband and my best friend. I can't
go through this alone. A load has been lifted, but my
heart still aches.*

This sharing brought us a little closer, and I found that, my
husband would be one of my most important resources through
my healing.

It is very important that a person has as many resources as
possible throughout their healing journey. Resources allow us
to keep moving with hope in times of desperation. Another
important resource for me included listening to K-LOVE radio
station. The words in the songs and those given by the broadcasters
soothe my soul. It seems that I always heard just the right song at
just the right time. I felt like they were playing a song just for me
many times throughout my healing, and I have no doubt the Holy
Spirit was the DJ. It is very important to surround yourself with
positive and encouraging elements to aid healing. This awareness
had removed a layer of pain in my arm and wrist, which I had
not previously been able release. This is an example of pain held
inside, which has expressed itself through body language. The
pain we hold in our heart and mind often finds a resting place
in the tissues of the body and sometimes comes back to haunt us
later, presenting itself as physical pain.

I began having more trouble sleeping. Insomnia had already
been a problem in my life for at least 15 years prior to this. I did
not know where I had gotten the energy to keep going for so
many years and be as active as I was with a business, 5 children,
and chronic daily pain. I would often be bragging proudly of
how I never slept but somehow was able to keep going. Others
would say, "I don't know how you do it!", and I took that as a

compliment. It inspired me to keep going. Over several months, I did begin to notice that something did not look right physically when I looked at myself in the mirror. Aside from the fact that I was constant pain, I thought I was fine. My mother, sisters and patients began asking me if I was feeling okay. It was obvious they saw something too. I began losing weight for unknown reasons. I started experiencing some nausea, and my eyes did not look clear. There was a haze over my eyes, like a film of rain over a glass. I had a very unsettling feeling that something was going to happen, and I was afraid of what it might be. Little did I know, these intuitive feelings would become reality.

CHAPTER 2

A Near Death Experience

On June 6, 2007, I chose to have an inter-scalene injection (a shot in front of the collar bone) to alleviate pain I had been having in my shoulder, thoracic spine and right arm for several years. I ignored the signs and symptoms my body had been giving me for so long to slow down. I wanted a quick fix so that I could keep going. I felt an obligation to take care of my family and all the patients who were in so much pain. During this injection, I lost consciousness, and perhaps lost my life for a brief moment. It was truly a near-death experience. As I lay there helpless, I saw a bright light and began to pray for God to spare my life. I was not ready to leave this life. My 11 year old daughter and 9 month old son were in the waiting room, and I had 3 other children at home, who needed me. I remember just asking the nurse to pray with me as I heard the doctor in the background yelling to "get the crash cart". The Hail Mary Prayer gave me great comfort, as well as The Lord's Prayer. As I said them over and over, I began to regain consciousness.

When I awakened, I could not feel or move my arms and legs. I quickly regained feeling and movement in my left side, but regained it much more slowly on my right side. I was terrified! What was happening? As I was elevated to an upright position, I began to faint again. I was unable to stabilize, so I was brought by ambulance to a nearby hospital. After evaluation by the physician, it was determined that I had a possible abnormal response of the vagus nerve to the injection, as well as anxiety. I was furious that they thought I had anxiety. I felt I had nothing to be anxious about: I had the perfect family, a job I loved, and a great sense of faith.

I was released and sent home with instructions to rest and return, if symptoms reoccurred. A few weeks went by and I was having some lightheadedness and a rapid heart rate. I had already chosen to stop working and focus on healing my chronic, degenerating back pain, which had been my constant companion for more than 20 years, and began taking care of my shoulder pain as well.

As I slowed down the pace of my life, it seemed my body came to a crashing halt. On June 26, I had another episode, which began with tremors in my legs, which eventually brought my body to a point of paralysis. I remember lying there conscious with my eyes closed and everything spinning around me, feeling paralyzed, and there was nothing I could do to stop it. It lasted several minutes, from what I can remember. I asked my husband to pray with me and to hold the calves of my legs, in order to calm my system. I learned this technique in one of the classes I attended. I was so thankful I had these resources, because they really helped to quiet my symptoms. I felt so alone and scared. I was having these episodes 1-2 times a week at this point. They would leave me extremely with no energy for hours. I had also noticed heart arrhythmias (skipped or abnormal beats) when I used my right arm or laid on my right side. As a result, I visited several doctors and had extensive testing. I was seen by a neurological cardiologist, who stated he was, "...99 percent sure that I had a blockage in the vertebral artery and that he could fix it with a stint." The MRI that was done showed no blockage, and everything appeared normal. The doctor was confused and speechless, and again I was sent home with instructions to rest and return if symptoms continued.

By this time, I was incredibly frustrated that no one could find an answer. I returned home and tried to resume normal activity, which, for me, consisted of going 90 miles an hour. I was very active and did not like to rest. All of a sudden, my body could not go like it used to. I noticed significant weakness on my right side, and I had a strong feeling I was having mini-strokes from blood clots. I submitted to more testing by several additional doctors, but nothing was found. I began to have more and more fainting spells, severe tremors and seizure-like episodes. I eventually ended up at a heart hospital, where I was diagnosed with vasovagal (sometimes called neurocardiogenic) syncope. Vasovagal syncope is described by the heart hospital as "...not a serious or life-threatening condition, but an abnormal reflex which results in a drop in blood pressure, leading to decreased blood flow to the brain, resulting in dizziness or fainting." I was so happy to have a diagnosis, but I still had no real answers as to why this was happening or had never happened before. How could I have gone from a perfectly healthy person, who had missed work once in the past 6 years, to being unable to drive, take care of my family and eventually myself. My only option was to take medication, which I never did well because of the odd sensations the drugs gave me. Also, I am a firm believer in the body's natural ability to heal itself. However, I gave it a try, since I had no other alternatives available at the time. I very quickly learned that this was not my answer, and I quit taking the medication. I knew there had to be some rational explanation for this. My next option was to have an ablation (burning) of the nerve to the heart, in order to make the symptoms stop. The heart doctor told me that if this did not work, I would need a pacemaker. I prayed and felt this was not my answer, so I decided to continue searching and receiving treatment from those who relieved my symptoms in a natural way. This is where I began to get answers.

CHAPTER 3

Spiritual Healing

All of a sudden, I began to experience fear like I had never known. I really dreaded the night time. The lack of sleep was getting worse, and I could not even nap during the day. My heart would wake me up, beating terribly hard and fast. I felt as though I had just run a race. I had to sleep upright in a chair for several months, if I was to get any rest at all. Lying flat would almost immediately start my heart racing. I returned to the hospital for a few more tests and wore a heart monitor for a month. I had several EKG's and an ultrasound. This only revealed that, yes, I had abnormal EKG's, but there was nothing else of significance to the doctors, so again, I was left without answers. Meanwhile, my dread was growing stronger. I tend to be a person 'in control', and I had a great fear of the unknown. I wanted answers, and I was not getting them. I grew weaker each day, and I had completely lost my appetite. I lost several pounds in a couple months time and my clothes swallowed me. It was often all I could do to force myself to eat a cracker and drink some water in the course of a whole day, because I knew I had to eat something to survive.

There were days I was so weak, my legs would collapse when I stood up, and my husband had to carry me to the bathroom. I was completely exhausted just by taking a shower. I had lost so much weight; I could see every bone in my body. I could no longer stand to look at myself. I woke up one night and looked in the mirror and I could not see the pupils of my eyes. This was one of the most fearful days of my life. Over the next few days, I looked and looked, and I still could not see my pupils. It was as if a glare and darkness was taking over. I asked my husband if he could see the pupils of my eyes, and he said, "Yes, why?" I was embarrassed and scared to share with him what I was going through, so I chose to keep it to myself.

I could not understand the terrors I was experiencing, and I wondered how God could let this happen. I was beginning to wonder what I had done wrong. I was doubting my faith.

I did have a few friends that I could talk to. They have been my ongoing strength throughout this journey. It was their treatments and prayers, as well as the prayers of many others, which kept me going. At this point in my healing, my greatest comfort was found in someone praying with me or over me, and in scripture. God, again, was there to give me strength. I would often call my dear friends, Margo and Vada, who are very gifted in prayer. They have been much needed resources, throughout my healing journey.

I began journaling letters to God. My first journal had a verse on the front that read "I *Am the Light of the World. Whoever Follows Me Will Never Walk In Darkness, But Will Have The Light of Life." John 8:12.* The scriptures gave me just what I needed each day. Through them, I found the strength and courage to continue on this journey. Journaling became yet another powerful resource for me. It was a tool that gave me direction in my healing, when all the roads I took seemed to have a dead end. I began to learn to ask for guidance and direction from God before attempting new testing or treatments. I've heard the song by Casting Crowns which says, *"The voice of truth tells you a different story..."* many times, but I really heard it's meaning during this time in my life. I began to understand the discernment of truth, as I journaled and really listened for answers and guidance through prayer. I have always prayed, but I never really slowed down long enough to see or hear the answers. We are so fortunate to have this gift. Why plant flowers, if we are not going to take the time to enjoy their beauty?

> JOURNAL ENTRY: 6-29-07 *Thank you Lord for all my wonderful family and friends. Their prayers are what are healing me through you. Thank you for the peaceful quiet times you are giving me just when I need them."* The verse on this page read: *"To the man who pleases Him, God gives wisdom, knowledge and happiness."* Eccles. 2:26. *I told my husband many times that I felt God was trying to show me something through all of this, not just for my healing, but for something greater he had in store for my life.*

CHAPTER 4

Emotional Blocks and How They are Connected to Physical Pain

The pain in my shoulder became so thick and so deep I lost feeling in part of my shoulder. The emotional part was not the only component of my pain. I did have physical injury in my shoulder from overuse and falls. These were corrected with surgery in August of 2007. However, the deep pain I experienced had not changed after my surgery. This was very frustrating. I found myself fighting a frozen shoulder for a year following my surgery.

Pain speaks to us, if we listen. Often, pain that stems from hidden emotional blocks may be described by the patient as a 'deep pain' that they cannot reach. The resulting physical feeling may be thick or even numb. When there is no trauma, and testing does not point to anything obvious, but the pain gets progressively worse over years, it can be associated with an emotion that has been buried. It may not have been the right time, or it may have been too painful to acknowledge. For these or other reasons, we may hide our emotional hurts to be able to function more effectively. This type of pain is often missed and is extremely difficult to diagnose and overcome, since all testing appears to be normal. This is often not understood in traditional medicine, and the exasperated patient is left without an answer and with the temptation to lose their hope.

Even though the root of the pain is emotional, it is often felt physically in the part of the body in which it was stored. We may wonder, why is God letting this happen? This does not mean that we have lost faith. Even Jesus cried out on the cross, saying, "My God, my God, why have You forsaken Me?" Matthew 27:46. When bad things happen, we have to remember that God may be trying to show us something or guide us to make a change in our life. Psalm 139:14 reminds us, "...*We are fearfully and wonderfully made...*". We are created in the image of God. When one area of our body is out of balance, all other systems of the body can be affected.

Have you heard the expressions 'shouldering a burden', 'something is eating at me', or 'I've got a load on my back'? If we really listen to our bodies, they give us the answers. It may not be spelled out or written in stone, but our symptoms will show us where to pay attention. It is an amazing gift to feel pain, because it gives us so many clues, as to what is really happening. Pain really is our friend, even though it seems like an enemy.

Can you imagine if we were not created to feel pain? Many would die from disease and cancer at a faster rate, because we would not have a signal alerting us that something is wrong and motivating us to seek the help we need. A spider bite could eat a hole through the back of a man's leg before he ever knew it was there. It is important that we address emotional pain when it comes our way, just as we do physical pain. Otherwise, it will find a place in our bodies to stay until we are ready to deal with it. The longer it is stored, the deeper it is buried, and the more layers of that onion we will have to peel in order to return to good health.

CHAPTER 5

More Answers and A Revelation

I continued to pray and journal, searching for answers. Looking back, I realize there were a great many layers of pain overlapping; it is no wonder we could find no answers through testing. Essentially, there was more than one answer, and I knew I had to keep looking. I felt strongly that God was trying to show me something. I found comfort in the verse, **"I am the resurrection and the life. He who believes in me will live, even though he dies."** **John 11:25**. At this point in my healing, I often heard the song by Matt Redman that says, "...*even though I walk through the shadow of the valley of death your perfect love is casting out fears......oh, no, you never let go, through the calm and through the storm.*" I walked through shadows in my valley that were so dark, sometimes I literally could not see.

> JOURNAL ENTRY: 7-19-07 *I feel so weak, my heart races, my heart pounds-this is so hard, I feel out of control-I know God is in control. I asked God to show me a sign of his healing today, and about 5 minutes later, Jacob (my son, who was eight at the time) walked*

up and put his hand on my head and said "God Bless You" then he did it again and said "I said a prayer for you, mom". Wow! What a sign! Thank you, God.

Physically, I was continuing to grow weaker. I was now in bed more than I was out of bed. The medicine I began taking for the shoulder pain was making me worse, so I began weaning myself off of it. I needed a lot of courage to keep my focus. Many verses gave me strength; Psalms 25:21, ***"May integrity and uprightness protect me, because my hope is in you"***, and Isaiah 41:10,***"Do not fear, I am with you, do not be dismayed, for I am your God. I will strengthen you and help you. I will uphold you with my righteous hand."*** My faith was deepening. It may not have appeared that way to many, because of my frustrations, but deep inside I knew God was trying to show me something and that he was going to give me answers. He was the one true physician I could count on in this time of despair.

JOURNAL ENTRY: 7-25-07 *Dear God, I trust you will tell me what I need to do. I feel so tired-so weak, I beg you to let my mind rest and keep me focused only on you and your healing for me. Keep my faith strong and don't let the devil interfere. Keep my loved ones strong- I need them so much right now but fear they are tired too. Help my husband and children stay strong- they move me forward every day, and I am so thankful you gave them to me. So, please, show me an answer for this pain-this trauma in my body.*

I was desperate for an answer, because I felt my days of surviving were numbered. ***Psalms 40:1: "I waited patiently for the Lord; He turned to me and heard my cry"***. It was not long after this cry for help that God gave me another answer. I woke up one night about 3:45 am, hearing what sounded like someone yelling the word "chelation" at me. I could not fall back asleep and the word chelation kept going through my head. What did this mean? I had heard the word before, and I knew it had something to do with cleaning toxins out of the blood. After being up the rest of the night, I was praying and asking God what this meant. I kept getting a metallic taste in my mouth, and it occurred to me that it might be mercury poisoning from the fillings in my teeth.

I anxiously waited until my husband woke up and told him about the dream I had. I was eager to find someone to test me for mercury poisoning. I called a doctor I knew and asked if she could test me for mercury poisoning. I told her that I felt God was leading me to an answer through my dream. She replied, "I don't think that is what God is telling you, but we can get you tested, if you want" I was grateful that she was willing to find a way to test me, but her comment left me disturbed. I had a strong sense that this was an answer to prayer, because I had told my husband a few weeks before this about a dream, in which I felt like there was something poisoning me from the inside, but I did not know what it was. I had asked him to promise me that he would keep searching, if I went unconscious, because I knew there was an answer. However, I did not know how much time I had left. I felt like I only had days, so I chose to go with what I thought God was showing me. I knew it sounded crazy to many, but I didn't care. I was certain there was truth in it. Isaiah 48:17 clearly states, ***"I, the Lord, your God, teach you what is for your good, and lead you on the way you should go."***

I once read in a devotion that guidance comes through prayer. We may not always feel like we know what to do. Our life may seem perfect one day, and shift like the wind the next. It is at these times that God leads us through personal prayer. By being patient and trusting in prayer, we may gradually receive little answers and see or feel the next step we need to take. Other times, God may lead us through scripture, through the eyes of our children, a comment from a friend, a story on the news, or even walking through a labyrinth. Someone once said, "The best spiritual director is life itself." God often uses the people and events in our daily life to teach us and lead us in the way we should go.

I continued to search for a test for mercury poisoning. No one could tell me just how I could get this done, so I consulted with a doctor I had heard of through a friend, who had nearly died from mercury poisoning from a flu vaccine. This doctor was a few hours away, and I suggested a phone consult. When I told him my symptoms, he said it was possible, but first he wanted me to do a 24-hour urinalysis to see if there might be something else going on. I got off the phone frustrated. I could not understand why it was so difficult to get such a simple test done. Why would no one believe me? Why did everyone try to blind me to what I had heard through the Holy Spirit? My best friend once told me, "Sometimes the closer you try to get to God, the more Satan tries to get to you". I have found so much truth in that statement throughout this journey. The beauty of it all is that the more I quiet myself and listen for God's word, the more I hear, and the easier it becomes to ignore the lies.

After speaking with my mother and sharing my frustrations, she reminded me of a doctor my father had seen, who had recommended IV treatments for my father's diabetes. She has always had a faith and trust in me, and she encouraged me to follow up with the tests for the heavy metal poisoning. She believed in me. At that moment, I remembered that it was in that same doctor's office where I had seen the pamphlets for chelation, Another answer from God. It is not a coincidence when we receive these messages at just the right time and place. Immediately, I called their office and asked to be seen. This doctor diagnosed me with adrenal fatigue and offered treatment with vitamin C and Oxidation IV treatments. I began to notice a difference with increased energy after the Vitamin C treatment. However, I would have arrhythmias during and after the oxidation treatments. The nurses providing the treatments would just add magnesium to the IV and tell me that it was normal.

After about a month of these treatments, I decided to insist on having a test for the mercury poisoning, because I still felt this is where God was leading me. He agreed to do the test, and finally it was confirmed. The test was a urinalysis using a chelating agent known as EDTA. Other testing for metals may use hair samples, saliva and electro-dermal screenings, which can be found more commonly through natural medicine or Naturopathic Doctors and some Chiropractors. My test showed not only significant levels of mercury in my blood but also aluminum and lead. The only source from which I knew I had mercury was my fillings. I have had nine of these fillings in my teeth, since childhood. I believe the aluminum was most likely from canned foods and from my deodorant, since that is the main ingredient in most deodorants. The lead was most likely something to which I had been exposed in the environment, since it is known that we are all exposed to lead-based paints throughout our surroundings.

After more research, I found information on the toxicity in silver fillings due to the mercury. I discovered that, when combined with aluminum, this toxicity is intensified, because of the molecular binding. I asked the doctor to do more IV treatments, in order to remove the metals from my blood. He agreed, and I began treatments.

As I received the treatments, I would notice an immediate difference. I could feel pressure being drawn from my right shoulder, my chest would tighten, my heart would beat fast, and then slow, and my eyes became clearer after each treatment. I felt like a new person for 2-3 days after each treatment. The brain fog and weakness would almost completely go away for a few days, but then it would return. It seemed that, when it returned, the symptoms became worse. In the meantime, I consulted with a holistic dentistry facility in Marble Falls, Texas and scheduled an appointment to have a dental revision done. A dental revision includes the removal of all dental metals and bacteria of the teeth. I found it is very important when removing silver fillings to have them removed carefully by a dentist, who knows what they are doing. The mercury being removed is extremely toxic. It is so toxic, in fact, that if mercury is removed incorrectly, it can be more harmful than if it were just left in the teeth. There is research showing that mercury toxicity is linked to many diseases including multiple sclerosis, lupus, cognitive disorders, and many more life-threatening illnesses. It is very likely that many deaths attributed to 'unknown cause' may be linked to various toxins in the body, 'the silent killers'.

Thank God he created such an awesome body. If our bodies could not take over and filter and eliminate the toxins we take in everyday, we would not survive very long. The body is truly amazing in its ability to heal itself, if we just listen to it and give it the time it needs.

After more questions and searching for answers, I found that I was becoming more toxic in some ways. The doctor providing the IV treatments had no answers for me. I consulted with the new dental facility I had found, and I was informed that chelation to remove metals from the blood should never be done until the fillings are removed, because the metals are pulled through the tissues; thus, the patient is made more toxic. I had to wait a few months before my revision; for this was the first appointment they had available. At this point, I felt I had to continue with the treatments at least once a week to keep me at a safe level, so I did. I was so sick and weak; I did not feel that I would make it if I completely stopped the treatments.

It was during times like these that I would become frustrated with the medical world. I would wonder why no one could provide me with the information I needed before it was too late. How could the medical world be so neglectful? Why did I have to find the answers? I slowly began to realize that it was not up to the medical world to give me answers. They can only guide me with what they know and the knowledge they have been given, which is often life-saving. I had to learn that I needed to give in to the will of God and not my own. It's easy to become angry and blame others for our transgressions, but what we have to realize is that God always provides us with what we need, if we just let Him. This is easier said than done, but it can be done. With constant prayer we will receive the answers we need. God will show us the truth if we truly listen.

After much anger, confusion, and frustration at the medical world, I began to be grateful for the answers I was receiving. The hardest part was the waiting. I found the more anxious I became about getting answers, the worse my situation became. I learned that part of my healing was giving in to the will of God and leaving it in His time, not mine. When I accepted this, my spirit received healing, and each day it became easier for me to face the physical and mental challenges I was having. God reveals all the answers we need, but if we interfere with His will and begin to rely on our will, sometimes we learn things that are not necessary or needed. If we force answers to come before God wants us to know them, we may find ourselves in a dangerous situation.

CHAPTER 6

Healing According to My Will

A perfect example of healing according to my will would be the shoulder surgery I rushed into in August of 2007. I had been suffering from this shoulder pain that only seemed to be getting worse, along with everything else I was going through. I had an MRI that showed a lot of inflammation with a possible rotator cuff tear, but the doctor with whom I consulted did not seem to think there was anything that needed to be done surgically. I consulted with another doctor, and again, she did not recommend anything be done surgically.

I searched on. I had so much pain; I knew there must have been something seriously wrong. Finally, I found a surgeon, who looked at my films and said I definitely needed surgery. He had me scheduled the next week. He gave me hope that maybe the shoulder problem was contributing to my heart arrhythmias. The surgeon had told me I had a labral tear in the shoulder, which was going to be a pretty significant surgery and recovery. I remember having 'that feeling' that this was not going to solve my mysterious shoulder pain and heart arrhythmias, but I chose to ignore it, because I was tired of waiting, and I wanted someone to 'fix me'.

I remember being prepped for surgery and thinking that maybe I should change my mind, but again, I chose to ignore it and went through with it. I remember waking up from the anesthesia with my heart racing and a distinct feeling that I was not safe, and that nothing had changed my heart or shoulder condition.

I came to find out I did not have a labral tear, so the surgery was not as extensive as we thought it would be. There was a small rotator cuff repaired, and I had a biceps tendon transfer, so my recovery should have been fairly quick, with full range of motion regained within a few months. I ended up much weaker after the surgery and had a frozen shoulder for the next year. The pain about which I had initially complained had not changed. In fact, it grew considerably worse. The doctor who did my surgery wanted me go back in for a second surgery, in order to release my frozen shoulder. He assured me it would be simple, and that I would have full range of motion as soon as he did the release. This time I prayed and listened to what God was telling me, and I chose not to go through another surgery. I was tempted, because it was very difficult living with a frozen shoulder, but I kept getting the message that it would take time and another surgery was not my answer.

> JOURNAL ENTRY 9-3-07: *Dear God, it's been a tough week. The surgery on my shoulder really weakened me. I feel so nauseous, tired and weak. I just want to be strong again. I want to be with my family-please help me get there. Thank you for my family's help. They sure have been there for me-help keep them strong. Help me eat and regain my strength. Help Doug (my husband) take one day at a time and not feel overwhelmed. Keep him and the kids healthy and strong.........may you reveal boldly what I need to get well. Psalms 147:3: He heals the brokenhearted and binds up their wounds.*

CHAPTER 7

Healing According to the Will of God

Once I found out the toxicity was coming from my fillings, I felt an urgency to have the fillings removed immediately. I could not understand how the dental facility could know how sick I was and not work me in right away.

While I waited for my dental appointment, I consulted with a naturopath. He informed me that I had severe adrenal fatigue and confirmed the heavy metal toxicity, as well as stressed areas of my body, including my liver, kidneys, and adrenal glands. By this point, my heart had become so weak that my blood pressure was dropping 30 points from a lying to a standing position. I would be out of breath from only walking 100 yards. Keep in mind, just a few months before this, I was able to easily walk 2-3 miles on my elliptical without getting tired. The naturopath immediately started me on some supplements to start rebuilding my strength. I began to eat and sleep again, but it was a very slow process. I was taking about 60 supplements a day and eating raw fruits and vegetables. It was the beginning of my road back to health.

I began to regain some strength. I had a difficult time getting the rest I needed, being at home with my husband and five children, so I prayed and made the very difficult decision to go stay with my parents for a few weeks. I think that was one of the hardest things I have ever had to do. At the time, my children were 14, 11, 8, 5, and 10 months. I had just recently had to completely stop nursing the baby, which was very difficult. The baby had a hard time being away from me, so it made my decision to retreat all the more difficult. I felt like my emotional heart was being ripped apart. Somehow, only through faith, did I feel that I was doing the right thing. I felt God was telling me to take this time for my healing, so I could one day take care of my family again.

JOURNAL ENTRY: 9-4-07: *Self-sacrifice not self-love*

JOURNAL ENTRY 9-21-07: *Dear God, I'm not sure what to feel right now. I miss my family- my husband and kids so much, and it is so hard being away from them. But I keep reminding myself these days will pass, and I will get stronger. I am so thankful for this time you are giving me to rest with my family- I am so blessed to have so many loving people around me- continue to guide me Lord and help me sleep so I can heal. I look forward to a better day tomorrow.*

JOURNAL ENTRY: 9-23-07: *Dear God, thank you for a better day. Thank you for time with my kids and husband. Thank you for the strength to let them go and trust I need this time away for healing. Help me to know when I am strong enough to return home. Help me learn to meditate/focus, whatever I need to shut down my brain for sleep and use that time to become closer to*

you Lord. I love you. "Jeremiah 29:13 "When you call
me, when you go to pray to me, I will listen to you."

I began to seek the face of God more and more. There was
some distress in this seeking, because, when I tried to imagine the
face of God, I could feel His presence and see light, but I could
not see His face. For this reason, I was driven to look harder and
more often. I found answers to this distress later in my healing.

By the time I went for my dental revision, I had gained the
strength I needed to survive the procedure. It was a blessing that
I was not able to get in for an appointment any sooner. I have no
doubt that I would not have been able to go through the revision,
if I had not first seen my Naturopath, Dr. Robbins. I had had no
idea what I was about to go through with my dental revision.
I thought it would be as simple as having my fillings removed
and replaced, like any other dental appointment. I was in for a
surprise. The procedure went well. I was under conscious sedation
for about 6 hours, although it seemed like an hour. Dr. Freeman,
the dentist who performed my revision, was very caring and did
a wonderful job. I felt very safe in her hands, and in the hands of
her staff in Marble Falls, Texas. Their prayers before they started
brought me much comfort. They not only removed the fillings
and replaced them with a resin that was compatible to my blood
chemistry (known through a biocompatibility blood test), but
they also opened and cleaned the area where my wisdom teeth had
been removed about 5 years before the revision. Lab results from
the dental revision later revealed there was a live bacteria living
in the pocket where my wisdom teeth had been removed. These
bacteria go into the bloodstream and are linked to heart disease
and autoimmune disease. I learned that it is very important when
a permanent tooth is pulled that it be pulled properly, by cleaning
the area thoroughly and suturing the area as it heals, so that none
of these life-threatening bacteria is left behind to haunt us later. A

helpful resource concerning this subject is the book <u>The Roots of Disease, Connecting Dentistry & Medicine</u>, by Kulacz and Levy. During the dental revision, Dr. Freeman reported that my heart rate remained elevated (96-102) even while under conscious sedation, which she found very unusual. After the revision, I immediately had a sense of improved health and safety. I actually had an appetite and wanted to eat for the first time in months. The haziness that was in my eyes almost immediately disappeared, the brain fog was at least 50% improved, the nausea was gone, and I had healthy color in my face again. I noticed immediately the pressure in my chest and heart arrhythmias were at least 50% better. My shoulder pain was very intense after the revision, which was explained as "the tissues trying to eliminate the metals". My urine had a strong metallic smell for the next 2-3 weeks.

JOURNAL ENTRY 10-16-07: (The day after my dental revision)

"Dear God, thank you for today. Thank you for helping me through this day with more laughter than tears, even with this pain. Lord help me to heal, if it be your will, help me to carry whatever cross I need-help me to remember you are there with me to hold any crosses I bear and to surrender completely Lord, to do your will, not mine. I will praise your name.

Within two days of coming home, I began to have severe headaches and whole body tremors. My temperature would fluctuate from 95.6 to 103.7. I would have tremors so bad throughout the day, that my whole body would ache from shaking so hard. It took all I had to remove my clothing when I wanted to get in a hot bath, because I was shaking so much. I would take 2-3 baths a day to calm the tremors and warm up. The tub would form a ring of a silver-white film after each bath for the next week. My headaches were non-stop. I was feeling like my head was going to explode, and nothing I did or took for the pain helped. I also had severe craniofacial pain. I did consult with a local physician, who said I had a urinary tract infection and wanted to put me on antibiotics, but I had a strong sense that this was part of the detoxing my body had to go through, in order to eliminate the metals. I had some doubt and filled the antibiotics prescription; however, I felt that struggle inside of me that told me it was not the right thing to do. I began listening closer to God's truth. A verse I read that week read, *"**Jesus said, 'Anyone who lets himself be distracted from the work I plan for him is not fit for the Kingdom of God.' Luke 9:62.***

There were many people, who would give me advice, and they all had good intentions, but I knew it was up to me to discern the truth that God was trying to show me. I needed to increase my faith and trust in the decisions I made. Romans 12:2 warns, ***"Do not conform yourself to this age, but be transformed by the renewal of your mind, that you may discern what is the will of God, what is good and pleasing and perfect".***

> JOURNAL ENTRY 10-21-07: *Dear God, sorry I have not written in a few days. I have been sick with fever since Friday. Thank you for the rest I have been getting. Please help me find the right resources to get rid of this pain in my right TMJ to my shoulder and my stomach pain. Please let me be able to eat better so I can gain some weight. Help me to take each day with a smile and never give up hope. Please let me be able to drive again soon to take the burden off my husband and others.*

CHAPTER 8

A Turning Point

By October 29, 2007, I drove a car for the first time in 4 months. By November 7th, 2008, I was driving independently again. I will never forget the day. I realized the freedom I had lost, and I found a new appreciation for the little things in life that we often take for granted. I had always been very independent, going wherever I needed to go, without a second thought. When I lost the ability to drive, I lost my freedom, and learned that the restriction was indeed a blessing. God was keeping me right where I needed to be, slowing down my life to once again "smell the roses". We must be grateful for each day, no matter what it brings. By October 30, 2007, I was able to stay home alone with my baby, Sammy, for the first time since June. I was very nervous, felt a little unstable, and was still having a lot of pain, but I will never forget the day. When I lost the ability to take care of my children, I was so angry. I could not understand how God could let me be so sick and give me these 5 beautiful kids that I could not care for. I had always felt it was my job to take care of the kids, to feed them, to bathe them, to do their laundry, the dishes, etc. I know we often get tired and complain about the daily chores we have in life, but when you lose the ability to do them, it makes you realize just how grateful we should be to have the health to do them. Instead of complaining about all the work I had to do, I now was grateful for each and every day I could do anything for the wonderful family God had given me.

I gained strength daily. However, the pain and loss of movement in my right shoulder persisted. I continued to have an elevated resting heart rate that varied from 104-120 beats per minute. During this season in my healing journey, I was receiving physical therapy for my back and shoulder pain. I noticed, after treatments to my shoulder, I would often have increased sympathetic nervous system responses, (rapid heart rate, nervousness, dizziness, arrhythmias, etc.) and the pain behind my right shoulder blade would increase. I had a palpable mass behind the right shoulder blade that did not change shape or size with physical therapy or massage therapy. It was often very sensitive to touch, and I could not tolerate any type of electrical stimulation on my body because it would cause heart arrhythmias and dizziness with an uneasy feeling.

This area of pain was a mystery and very frustrating to live with. I was hopeful that as I was detoxing from the metal poisoning, the mass and pain in the shoulder would go away, but I had a feeling that there was more to my story. I had a sense that God was trying to show me something more, and for some reason, I was very scared to see what might be coming. I am a kinesthetic learner. I learn best by experiencing a situation, and I wanted to continue to gain the knowledge God was giving me, because I knew He would use it for His good. There were many times I prayed for it to stop, because I didn't know how much more I could take. I have always been told that God never gives us more than we can handle, but I sure felt I was at my limits.

CHAPTER 9

A Renewed Strength

I had owned my business for 6 years, and I had not been aware of the stress I was letting myself carry. As far as performing the therapy, there was no stress other than wanting to "fix" everyone. I know, without a doubt, that giving therapy is a gift, and I absolutely love what I do. It was trying to keep up with all the business aspects that brought me much stress. I realized that I was trying to do it all. My mother always said, "You can't do two jobs and do them both well". I never intended to have a private practice; it just seemed to happen over time. I had many thoughts on giving up my practice, because I was exhausted with trying to keep the billing current to make enough income to keep the practice running. It seemed we were working so hard as therapists, doing quality work with such compassion for our patients, yet we were often having to fight to be compensated for our work. It truly took the passion out of what I had spent so many years training to do. I soon realized that I had to let go of the control I thought I needed and start trusting others to do the job I was not created to do. I am so thankful for the staff at Quality Physical Therapy. If it were not for them keeping things running while I was ill, there would be no Quality PT today. I was forced to delegate duties to others and trust that it would be okay. I no longer had the energy to do it all. This was a very important transition in my practice. I knew I either had to give it up or give up the control. I did a lot of praying and journaling and God brought me what I needed to keep Quality PT going. I was able to let go of another large layer of pain I had been carrying in my shoulder.

Making changes in my business in order to eliminate the stress, I began to feel more peace in my life. I recovered mobility in my shoulder but noticed I had significant weakness of my right side. I became aware that I was slumping a lot on my right side and had frequent dazed spells. I would often have increased occipital headaches after therapeutic release of my right shoulder. I asked God once again, through prayers and journaling, to guide me to healing. Ask, and you shall receive!

> JOURNAL ENTRY 11-24-07: Asked *Doug not to go hunting-feeling unstable. My heart feels like it's going to stop. I can't stop crying. I want to be be with Doug and the kids. I love them so much. Lord please guide Dr. Black's hands today. Thank you for all you have taught me. Help me to take one day at a time. Help me see what you are showing me. Help me accept what you are giving me. Lord, take me, if it is your will. Give me hope, if it is not. I love you and will praise your name no matter what.*

I kept telling my husband that I had the sensation I was throwing blood clots somewhere in my right shoulder area, because I would have the feeling that blood was being cut off to my head and my heart. It seemed to always happen with movement or use of my right arm. I mentioned it to a few doctors, and a few tests were done, but nothing showed up. So we continued to search for answers.

> JOURNAL ENTRY 11-25-07: *Lisa did some neural biofeedback yesterday and today. It seems to be helping. What an amazing body you made us Lord. My heart rate was 78 after treatment today. My sleep has not been good the past two nights. Please help me sleep better tonight and each night ahead. Help the waves in my brain to balance. Help me to regain control of my body. Help me to know my limits and not fear what is happening in my body. If any part of my healing needs medical attention guide me to the right person/place. Thank you for each day with my family.*

I did not really know the benefits of the neural biofeedback I was receiving at the time, but months later it would prove to be a great part of my healing. I knew it would help my overall brain function, but I did not understand why I was having these symptoms in my brain, or why nothing was showing up on any diagnostic testing. All I knew was that it felt like the right thing to do, and that I met Dr. Black at a crucial time, it was no coincidence.

I began to be amazed with all the wonderful people and new areas of healing that God was showing me. It was during this time that I realized that my learning was greater than my suffering. The fear of the unknown became less, and I began to feel a calmness I had not known before. My trust and faith in my answers were deepening. My spirit was healing in a way I never knew it needed.

Seeing Dr. Black for neural biofeedback I began to regain some brain function which I had lost. The ability to concentrate and organize was returning, the tremors decreased, and my heart rate began to stay at a more normal rate even when I had episodes. I also began to experience longer, deeper sleep which is very important in healing. I once again began to feel like 'the old Susie'.

JOURNAL ENTRY 12-5-07: *Another day to be thankful for. Thank you God for helping me make the most of it. I get frustrated with my limitations but I look at how far I have come and I am so thankful. Lisa is really helping to calm down my central nervous system and in the process I have learned something new once again. I am learning to express my feelings. I have kept my deepest emotions to myself all my life. Lisa asked at my last session, "How do people really know you, if you don't share your feelings?" I never thought of it that way. I did not mind sharing the good things in my life, but I had become an expert at hiding the tears and difficult times in my life. It occurred to me that is important in all aspects of my life-my relationship with my husband, friends, family, and my work! Thank you God for another valuable learning experience.*

CHAPTER 10

Spiritual Healing

If you have never read <u>Celebration of Discipline, The Path to Spiritual Growth</u>, by Richard J. Foster, you must put it on your list. My friend, Dr. Lisa Black, gave me this book not long after we met. It was just what I needed at this time in my life. My spirit needed healing. This is a part of who we are that we tend to disregard and it is so important in any healing experience.

I began to realize how important it was to be able to express my feelings and share them. I wondered how I could have known my husband for 20 years, yet I still could not share my deepest feelings with him. I began to wonder if he really knew me, or if I even knew myself. I had been trained at an early age (in-utero) to keep the bad stuff inside. I saw it as a weakness to complain of pain. Instead I would boast of all I was able to do, in spite of my daily pain. I thought I was a 'tough person' for being able to continue each day with a smile, even though I was crying on the inside. The smiling was mostly shown outside of my home, at work, to friends, etc. When I would arrive home from work most days, I would be in tears or in a rage that seemed uncontrollable. I was not angry at anyone at home, but it was the only way I knew to express myself and let go of the pain I was holding in. This led to many arguments with my husband and many regrets for the way I spoke to my children. Little did I realize what a poor example I was setting. I was showing my children to react to negative situations just the way I did, as did many generations before me. Because of my foolish pride, I had refused to ask for help. Instead, I had caused more suffering to come upon me physically, emotionally and spiritually.

> JOUNAL ENTRY 12-12-07 : The *skipped beats came back yesterday. Yesterday was a difficult day. I had a lot of dizziness- I had one dizzy spell that actually made me start to fall over. I had some nausea and loss of words. The pain still comes and goes and so does the detox symptoms (strong urine, disorientation, etc). Today is a little worse- I woke up early with tremors and crying-I still feel dizzy. It is so frustrating not knowing a definite answer. I get tired of being my own doctor, no doctor gives me guidance, none can give me an answer. God, you are the ultimate physician- you know the reasons for my pain, my anxiety, my depression, my dizziness, my increased heart rate, my chest pressure, my lack of range of motion. Please reveal an answer- I need to move forward.*

CHAPTER 11

Emotional Healing

Again, ask, and you shall receive! Six months of the unknown and many tears later, I was still posing as a warrior. My husband would often ask if I needed anything, and I would simply answer, "No, I'm fine". Deep inside, I wanted to cry out to him, but I did not know how to make him understand what I was feeling, and that I desperately needed him at this time. I felt so alone and scared at times, I just needed him to understand. Well, one day he brought home an article from a friend, who also had an ill wife. The article was called *"You Don't Look Sick"*. It was a true story of a young girl living with an auto-immune disease, which caused a great many limitations in her life. She appeared healthy on the outside; therefore, very few people knew how she really felt. She went on to explain, in detail, her struggles in life, so that her friends could understand the reality of what was going on in her body. I was in tears by the middle of the story, because it was just what I needed to help my husband understand just a fraction of what I was going through each day. I knew, for the first time since I became ill, that he understood, in some small way, just what I was feeling, and that I did really need him and his understanding to help me get well. We became closer in our relationship at this point, and I was able to share a little more with him each day. A tremendous amount of stress was taken from me, as I learned and allowed myself to open my heart to him. We learned several months later that listening was one key in our relationship, which we were not using very well when communicating. (chapter 21)

Always remember, if you are ill or just going through a difficult time in your life, do not try to handle it yourself. Talk to your best friend, which is hopefully your spouse, if you are married. Accept help when it is offered, and ask for it when it is needed. It is not a weakness that we cry out for help, but an acceptance of God's grace. We will all be stronger, in the end, for accepting this gift. The weakness actually lies in being too prideful to ask for help. God's strength is revealed in our weakness- all Bible heroes are examples of this.

Sharing these emotions seemed to ease some of my symptoms. Although I had the dizziness, the heart arrhythmias, and the fatigue, I learned that keeping the emotions inside actually intensified my symptoms. I once read that stress is actually the deadliest disease in America. It is important to learn to manage your stress and be aware of the signs of stress. Many will deny they are ever under any stress, because they do not even realize it themselves. It is helpful to have your husband or a close friend to hold you accountable. Ask them to help by telling you when they notice any signs of stress. Some of those signs may be fatigue, chronic illness, poor sleep, poor attitude, lack of motivation, inability to concentrate, etc. Other helpful suggestions may include documenting/journaling symptoms you may have and what makes them better, worse, how long they last, what time of day/year they happen, if you notice a pattern in response to food you have eaten or people you are around, etc. Keep these documents/journals and read back over them when you experience the symptoms.

A few days passed after the sharing with my husband, and we continued to pray for answers. It was the first week of December, 2007. We were going to buy some goat's milk and eggs from our neighbor. We started discussing my health issues and they were nice enough to offer to do a detox ionic footbath. These are used to eliminate toxins from the body. I had had some footbath treatments in the past, which seemed to help, so I accepted. I felt very strange sensations pulling from my head down my chest and right arm as the foot bath was going. The bath had colors of white, orange and black flecks which are signs of lymphatic waste, joint waste, and metals. I felt an immediate relief of pressure from my heart. The next day my journal read:

> JOURNAL ENTRY 12-10-07: *Today is the first day I have not noticed a skipped beat in my heart since June. My heart rate is still ranging from 84-104, but it is not as noticeable or distressing. I also have not coughed as much since the foot bath. The pain behind my shoulder is still intense but not as frequent today. Thank you, God, for the progress.*

Three days later I had a return of pain in my right arm, increased odor of my urine (usually a sign of detoxing), increase daze spells, and decreased memory.

> JOURNAL ENTRY 12-14-07: *A lot of pain in thoracic spine T2-T4. Pain is sharp/deep/stabbing/ burning. Feels like blood supply is being cut off. Feels like squeezing on my wrist and stiffness/pain in the fingers of my right hand, mostly upon wakening.*

> JOURNAL ENTRY: 12-17-07: *Prayed for more answers. Woke up with strong feeling of possible blood*

clots/arterial blockage-confirmed with blood in my urine-looked just like foot bath.

This was a dream like the one I had about my answer for the metal poisoning. I knew God was trying to show me something. This was an answer; however, it was not confirmed until a year later (Chapter 20). I know there were reasons that the answers were not revealed right away. God has a perfect time for everything, and he only shows us what we need to see when we need to see it.

The next day, December 18, 2007, I had an appointment with my naturopathic doctor for a three month follow-up. I told him what I had experienced with the blood in my urine and foot baths and told him that I felt I had blood clots that were causing an arterial blockage. He listened but did not seem too concerned. He thought that it might be referred pain from the liver detoxing so he decided to change my supplements. It is common for problems in the liver to cause referred pain in the right shoulder. It made sense, but I was frustrated that he was not as concerned as I was about the possibility of blood clots.

As I used the ionic foot bath 1-2 times a week through April of 2008, I kept notes of my results following each treatment. The foot baths had blood clot material, lymphatic waste and black metal flecks. I had relief of symptoms 2-3 days after each treatment which gave me the sense that the foot baths were keeping me safe, at the same time I knew there was more to the story. I had the impression that I had a life-threatening condition, but that God would keep me safe until it was time for an answer.

On January 7, 2008, I did follow up with a heart doctor to rule out any heart condition. He felt the problem was mechanical in nature, which means that the body may have an obstruction due to injury or lack of movement somewhere so he ordered an MRI of my thoracic spine. By January 23, 2008, I received results of the MRI. It was revealed that I have a large herniated disc of the thoracic spine at level T6-T7. The MRI report stated that CSF (cerebral spinal fluid) flow was void at that level. Again, I was thankful that more answers were revealed, and I thought this may be where part of my blood flow was being blocked. Two surgical opinions later, I had no good answers. Both surgeons told me I had a very complicated case with my heart symptoms and did not leave me much of an option other than to live with it. A thoracic disc herniation is very uncommon and very dangerous on which to perform surgery. One of the surgeons recommended a discogram of my cervical spine to rule out disc disease that may be causing my pain and then some nerve blocks of the thoracic spine to help the pain. Once these were done, he said he would consider a surgery. As much as I wanted someone to just fix it, I knew it was not that easy. I prayed for the right answer and God showed me that this was not my answer. Discograms are very stressful to the body and I did not want to numb the pain only to cause more injury, I wanted my pain to give me an answer, and this was not it. I kept seeing an image of God's hand on my back, and I knew He was going to be the one to heal me. I chose to continue with prayers, physical therapy, foot baths, neural biofeedback and nutritional supplements. I was progressing with my strength and energy but the heart arrhythmias continued to be a problem, as well as my revved up nervous system. It seemed I was having more trouble sleeping again, and I was having sensations of anxiety and depression.

> JOURNAL ENTRY 2-6-08: *Ash Wednesday,*
> *Thank you for helping me through this fast today- for*
> *replacing my hunger with your strength. I asked for a*
> *message from you and opened the Bible to the book*
> *of Mark and you gave me these words "Abba Father,*
> *for with you all things are possible, remove this cup*
> *(suffering) from me, yet not what I want, but what you*
> *want" (Mark 14:36). Teach me to pray, as you did.*
> *Give me strength to overcome my despair. Give me faith*

to abandon myself in God's hands, as you did. Give me
hope to see a new life beyond these moments of pain and
hopelessness. Amen.

Have you ever tried to fast? Do you know the benefits of
a fast? Do you think it is for weight loss? For cleansing? For
emotional/spiritual healing? Yes! It is for all of the above. There
are many ways to fast. You should always seek the advice from a
healthcare professional when attempting a fast. Times we need to
fast may be for pain, fever, illness, after surgery or dental work
or after traumatic injury. Times we may chose to fast may be for
general health, before a long airplane trip, for spiritual/emotional
healing, to heal chronic disease or to lose weight. We should not
fast if there is extreme liver congestion, low electrolytes, if on
an extreme acid diet, when not emotionally prepared, when you
cannot physically or emotionally rest while fasting or if you have
cancer. There are some exceptions with cancer. Otherwise, a fast
is very safe and effective when done under the care of a healthcare
professional.

You may be wondering how a fast can help emotionally and
spiritually. The reason is because the body does not have to work
so hard using energy to digest food. Fasting causes re-activation
of symptoms whether they be physical, emotional, or spiritual.
Therefore, it is very important that you have a positive attitude
and are ready for unexplained depression and irritability while
fasting. It is an amazing healing experience!

CHAPTER 12

Generational Curses

What is a generational curse? I am not speaking of any kind of witchcraft when I speak of curses. I am talking about those areas in our life that cause us to struggle physically, emotionally or even spiritually. An example of a physical generational curse may be a heart defect, cancer, cleft palate, or a congenital hip deformity, just to name a few. Emotional curses may be a result of the attitudes we carry which we learned or inherited throughout our lifetime. Spiritual curses are carried in our soul. This is the deepest part of our being. If our soul is at peace, the rest is easy. Spiritual and emotional curses may sometimes be at a subconscious level. Therefore, we may not be aware of why we act or react in a certain way to certain situations.

We often have 'a sense' that something is not right or that something may have happened in our past that is affecting us now, but it is often difficult to believe it. Some of us choose to look deeper, while some of us chose to look the other way. It is not easy facing our fears, but if you are willing, the process may help you to know and believe in who you are and who you were created to be. One of my favorite sayings is, "If God brings you to it, he will bring you through it."

I began to understand the term 'generational curse'. During mass, one Sunday Father Wilbur Moore's sermon was on spiritual generational curses. My journal reads:

> JOURNAL ENTRY 2-10-08: *Generational Curse"- There's that phrase again. Father Moore talked about spiritual generational curses today. We can blame others, or we can take responsibility and change the way we live. Life is what you make it. So now I have seen and lived how it applies to a person-physically, emotionally and spiritually. These are the answers I have received through my healing- I prayed for a way to help my family at more than a physical level, because I could see, but worse, feel the deeper level of their pain. Thank you God for all you have shown me. Help me to use it for good-for your will, not mine.*

CHAPTER 13

Guidance Through The Holy Spirit

I was not aware that I would soon be facing a deeper revelation in and about my life that would truly teach me the meaning of spiritual, physical and emotional generational curses. My life would be changed forever. I would finally begin to understand just who I am.

> JOURNAL ENTRY 2-27-08: *Thank you Lord for more answers, more pieces to my puzzle. My hormone test revealed significant deficiencies in many areas, especially cortisol which comes from adrenal insufficiency-then there is low progesterone, estrogen and testosterone, and decreased thyroid, which explains many of my symptoms. There is that 'generational curse'. I see my whole family affected and suffering from it. Help me continue to grow stronger and wiser so I can help them through your works. Please complete the pieces of my*

puzzle. I am so anxious to share what I am learning.
Help me to know my limits and to do your will not mine.

These results were just one more piece to my healing puzzle.
I am thankful for the knowledge I already had about hormones.
I had done a lot of reading in the past because of hormonal
symptoms I had. When I was 33, I consulted with my OB-
GYN about problems I was having which included insomnia,
irritability, dryness, fatigue, loss of hair and many more. I was told
at this time that I was "premenopausal" I was put on a synthetic
estrogen and told that it would take care of my symptoms. This
led to worse symptoms and I missed my period for 3 months.
My body was really confused. I began to read a book a friend
had recommended, <u>Women's Bodies, Women's Wisdom,</u> by
Catherine Northrup, and I began to find answers there. I returned
to having normal periods but continued to have many of the same
symptoms, the worse being insomnia. Another good reference
for hormonal imbalance is <u>Menopause, What Your Doctor May
Not Tell You About Pre-menopause : Balance Your Hormones
and Your Life from Thirty to Fifty</u> by John R. Lee, M.D., Jesse
Hanley, and Virginia Hopkins.

Like any other disorder, there are many reasons for hormonal
imbalances. Our hormones are affected by what we eat, how
we live, decisions we make, emotional blocks, stress, genes and
many more. In a perfect scenario, if we ate a naturally right diet,
had no stress, and lived our life according to the will of God, we
would have no menopausal or peri menopausal symptoms. Our
so called 'change of life' would be just that, a change in our life
that is natural as we grow older.

We are initially blessed with hormones at the time of
conception. Depending on our conception this may be the
beginning of a strong neuro-endocrine system, as God designed,
or a dysfunctional one that will need strengthening. Dr. Mines
quotes in her book <u>Pre and Perinatal Psychology</u>. "We have

the capacity to learn from and remember our prenatal lives and our births. These events get translated via hormones and other messengers into an indelible biologic blueprint that impacts us at some level for the rest of our lives, says Dr. Christine Northrup." Further, she quotes, "Every emotion and biochemical change associated with emotion in parents affects development from conception onward. Changes in stress hormones, such as cortisol and epinephrine create neuro-chemical cascades that shape immune function and health." The way in which a child is conceived and the situation surrounding that conception make a profound difference in the development of that person and how they will react to situations throughout their lifetime. We interfere with God's unique design when we do not conceive in love or allow a child to be born in His time; by this I mean pre-planned c-sections or inductions. There may be times when it is medically necessary, but not just because the doctor is going out of town or because we have company scheduled at a certain time to help. Just one day, even one minute, truly makes a difference.

When a married man and woman conceive a child in love, the foundation is laid for a nervous system that functions as God designed. Yes, there are genetic predispositions that may change DNA and generational issues that may pass to the child from the mother or father, but this type of conception will usually give a strong foundation to this new life. With this said, we can see and understand the importance of following God's plan for the gift of sex in marriage. From the beginning, God commanded in Genesis 1:28, ***"Be fruitful and multiply, and fill the earth and subdue it; and have dominion over the fish of the sea, and over the birds of the air, and over every living thing that moves upon the earth.***

Unplanned/unwanted pregnancies can weaken the foundation of a developing nervous system and lead to poor functioning of the neuro-endocrine system. Unnatural forms of birth control all contribute to disruption of a women's natural cycle therefore altering hormone levels which can ultimately be related to a poor functioning nervous system. Natural Family Planning (NFP) not only allows you to know your body but provides a natural way of conceiving or spacing while strengthening your marriage. There are no side effects and it is 99% effective. The only three 100% effective methods of birth control are abstinence, removal of the ovaries, or removal of both testicles. If we simply follow God's plan of the sex and marriage covenant, we can change the world one life at a time. If you are interested in more information on this you can find it at The Couple to Couple League for Natural Family Planning, Creighton Model of NFP by Pope Paul VI Institute, and the Billings Method.

Blood tests were done to check my hormone levels; they showed normal results although my symptoms told me different. I decided to do a saliva test to check my hormone levels and this gave me a whole different story. My results showed significant low levels of estrogen, progesterone and testosterone. I also had significant low levels of cortisol which confirmed I had a severe case of adrenal fatigue. You are probably wondering why the blood test did not show these results. I asked the same questions and found a logical explanation. Our blood is constantly being filtered in order to allow the body to get rid of waste and toxins, therefore our red blood cells die and regenerate about every 90 seconds which is why results may be inaccurate. A more accurate blood test can be done through what is called a "live cell" blood test which checks capillary blood versus blood serum. This test is done by taking a person's blood and immediately examining it under a dark field microscope. The saliva test shows a more accurate picture of what is going on in the body, because it is shows the amount of hormones that are actually available to be used by the cells; whereas traditional blood tests show all hormones circulating in the blood whether or not they are usable to the cells. Some hormones bind to proteins and may not be accessible because of deficiencies or toxins in the body, so even though they show up in a blood test, they are not being used. We need to see what is actually being used by the body. A fair analogy would be a basketball team. Say you have 12 people on a team, and 6 of the players show up to practice but are too sick to play. They may be present, but they are of no use to the team. This leads one to ask more questions. Why are my hormone levels too high or too low? The answer is not, "It's a normal part of the aging process". True, we may be aging, but what we really need to look at is what we may be doing wrong or may have done wrong in the past to get to this state of ill-health.

It is not always necessary to take hormone replacement supplements, because we can regain normal levels by changing our lifestyle in various ways, such as eliminating stressors, eating more healthy foods, and eliminating toxins. However, there may be an appropriate time to use hormone replacement therapy. If the hormone levels are so depleted that the body cannot obtain sleep or gain enough energy to make the right changes, then it is time to try hormone replacement therapy. It is important that the hormones are natural, compounded, preferably trans-dermal to obtain optimal results. There are many hormone supplements available that are synthetic in nature which are not as effective, because our bodies not only have to eliminate the synthetic byproducts, but the percentage that actually gets used by the cells is very minimal. Natural hormone replacement therapy and testing kits can be found at a compounding pharmacy or through a healthcare professional.

I had made many changes in my lifestyle, did much detoxifying from the heavy metal, and was eating quite healthy I was still having much difficulty sleeping, and this was keeping me from getting well. I decided to start using natural hormone replacement therapy, and I immediately began sleeping better. I truly had forgotten what it felt like to get a good night's sleep, and I did not realize how sleep-deprived I had been for the past several years.

My whole family appeared to have the same problems as far as hormonal imbalance just in different areas. Some of us suffered from low progesterone, high or low estrogen, low testosterone, low thyroid, increased or decreased cortisol levels. This had been a mystery I wanted more answers to since it had affected all of us in different stages of our lives. I had noticed our children's hormone imbalances had became more apparent at an earlier age.

The hormone creams were helping and my sleep improved, but it was not steady. I would often have nights with elevated pain behind my right shoulder, the immense pressure on my chest, and increased arrhythmias. I felt that the hormones were something I needed at this point, but God was trying to show me why. This hormone depletion made a significant impact on my body's ability to heal my many ligamentous joint problems. In the meantime, I had found a wonderful doctor in Tulsa, Dr. Weldon, who was providing prolotherapy treatment for the healing of pain syndromes. Prolotherapy is a type of therapy that is more complimentary in nature, therefore it is not heard of as much as it should be. It involves a series of injections using a proliferant to stimulate re-growth of ligaments and cartilage.

> JOURNAL ENTRY 3-28-08: *Had prolotherapy by Dr. Weldon - 174 injections to the lumbar and SI area. Very painful first 24 hours, back straight, and minimal to no pain after 24 hours. Spinal headache within 12 hours-so painful and debilitating-I'm on day 3, I can barely stand it. I heard you say, Lord, "I will walk by faith even when I cannot see. This brokenness brings your will for me." Thank you Lord for sustaining me - give me strength to get through this - carry this cross for me.*

> JOURNAL ENTRY 4-3-08: *The headache still lingers but I am getting better. I feel changes in my*

> *central nervous system. I know God is healing me. My treatment with Micha and Margo this week was profound - the balancing/change in my heart rhythm and central nervous system. I asked for a message today. I got my answer in Luke 6:42: "How can you say to your neighbor,' Let me take out the speck in your eye.' when you yourself do not see the plank in your own eye. You hypocrite, first take the plank out of your eye, then you will see clearly to take the speck out of your neighbor's eye." I take this as a message to take care of myself and stop trying to help others in areas that God has not called upon me. I struggle with giving God control to help my family- I see their hurts, pain, suffering, and I want to help- I become frustrated, my heart stressed-I give it to you Lord- may your will be done for my family, not mine, use me as you wish.*

I began to realize just how much pain and suffering I had absorbed while treating others. I realized that God was trying to show me that this healing was not mine, but His. I thrived from the compliments and statements of others after treatments. I needed constant praise and approval that what I was doing was helping others. I would get very distressed if someone did not respond well to the therapy I was providing. I always felt like I did not provide something I should have, and my thoughts would torture me. I would often take this stress home and continue to think of what I could have done better. In exploring what the Lord would have me do, I began to understand what God was showing me. I realized it was not my job to 'fix' people, and that the glory belonged to God, not me. I have a gift that God has given me, and I was abusing it. My intentions were good, but I was trying to fix everyone I thought I should without first asking permission or waiting for God to bring them to me. I was interfering with what God was trying to work through others and trying to take control of their healing. As much as my focus was on returning to work, I knew I needed to heal myself first. I needed to 'practice what I preach', in order to be a better example to my patients.

In order to rest and regain strength, I let go of responsibilities at my office that were burdening me and allowed myself to trust the wonderful person God had sent to manage my office. This had been a problem I had had in needing to control everything around me. I always felt the need to dictate and manage situations concerning my life and business, but I soon realized I could not do it all. This is where I began to trust and believe that God would take care of it. Trust was something that was not instilled in me as a child, rather, the opposite was learned. No one was to be trusted and if something seemed too good to be true, it probably was. Many of us grow up learning things from our parents, grandparents, siblings, etc., but it does not mean we are doomed to continue with that pattern in our life. This is part of an emotional generational curse. This is where our faith can help us to discern truth: do we continue patterns of learned behavior, or do we trust that God will show us what we need to do and where we need to be? This can and will have a profound effect on future and past generations, because the person that follows God has peace, and he or she carries that special light within them. They are envied by all who pass by them. There is no greater example. This was something I desperately wanted.

> JOURNAL ENTRY 4-23-08: *Thank you God for this awesome day. Thank you for the energy to clean my house, to take care of my kids, to cook healthy meals. Lord, thank you for all the resources you give me. Thank you for my wonderful husband. May you strengthen us together in your love each and every second of everyday. Thank you for allowing me to care for my children again. Help me to know their needs and to help them to be a*

> *healthy as they can possibly be and especially to guide*
> *them to know you Lord, to love you and live for you.*
> *Thank you for the rest you give me, help me to continue*
> *to know my limits. Guide me in all the right decisions*
> *of my practice. Continue to guide me to the resources I*
> *need for healing, physically, spiritually and emotionally.*

God led me to more answers. I was seen by an orthopedic
surgeon, who took some simple x-rays of my hips, which showed
I had a congenital hip dysplasia (a partial dislocation of the hip
since birth). This was big news for me. I finally could understand
where the feeling of instability in my back had been coming from
for the past 20 years. I had x-rays of my hips previously, but it
was never found. Obviously, it was not something God wanted
revealed until now. Finding all this, I had a sense of peace, for
the first time in many years, that I would need surgery, and that
we had finally found the source of my back pain, scoliosis and
degeneration. Unfortunately, it was not that easy. This surgeon
was more concerned with my back, because of the significant
degeneration and disc disease I had developed, and he was sure I
would need a back fusion before he would touch my hip. I left his
office very frustrated and confused, because I had fought the back
fusion for many years. I did not feel the surgery was my answer. I
knew God must be trying to show me something else.

I met a new physician referred to me by my dear friend, Dr.
Lisa Black. Dr. Prise is a very unique physician, who was very
caring and interested in my unique health issues. He provides
hyperbaric oxygen therapy to assist in healing by providing
restored oxygen to the cells. I felt very comfortable and led to
meet with him, so I did. The oxygen treatments did not appear
to be what I needed at the time but more importantly he was able
to make me aware of some other things. He showed me that my
heart arrhythmias, shoulder pain and chest pressure seemed to be
tied to something I feared. I began to ask God to show me what

this fear might be, and to help me face it rather than run from it, because I knew it was going to be another great component of my healing.

During this time, I had a dream that was so peaceful. I felt the presence of God so close in the midst of such a beautiful light, I felt his healing touch. This dream was my message telling me it was going to be okay, and not to give up, because God would be there to help me through, no matter what this fear was. In some ways, I was very anxious to find the answers, and I knew it had a enormous spiritual and emotional connection to my healing. On the other hand, I was terrified because of the deep emotions and tremors I began to experience.

My days began to be filled with endless crying. I was experiencing such a deep emotional pain; I could not stop the tears. I found it difficult to take care of and be around my husband and children. I did not want them to see me crying, or to see the intense pain I felt inside of me. These emotions overwhelmed me. My husband did not understand and was becoming very concerned. I needed his support more than ever, but I did not know how to share with him what I could not understand myself. Sharing emotions is not something I believed was good and natural. I had learned that to hold it in was better and perhaps easier than letting someone see you were crying. I saw emotions as a weakness, so I did not know how to share them. But at this point, I had to share, or I was concerned that I might go crazy. I gained relief with Psalm 69:2-4, 7-10 that says *"Save me God, for the waters have reached my neck, I have sunk into the mire of the deep, where there is no foothold, I have gone down to the watery depths, the flood overwhelms me. I am weary with crying out, my throat is parched. My eyes have failed, looking for my God. Let those who wait for you not be shamed through me, Let those who seek you not be disgraced through me. For your sake I bear insult, shame covers my face. I have become and outcast to my kin, a stranger to my mother's children. Because zeal for your house*

consumes me, I am scorned by those who scorn you." These words were profound to me, and I knew I would need greater strength and support than ever to face what God was about to show me.

I decided to cancel further appointments with Dr. Prise and focus on what God was trying to show me regarding these fears and emotions. I knew I had to heal emotionally before even considering a surgery.

> JOURNAL ENTRY 5-11-08: *Dear God, it's Mother's Day and I am so thankful you allow me to be here with my family. To be a proud mother of 6 (I only had five at the time! I did not know about a year later I would be pregnant with #6. I am not sure if I wrote 6 because of the twin I lost with Sammy or because somewhere inside God was showing me we would have another child) and the wife of a husband I love. I ask a lot of him but feel I need more. I don't feel close to him in ways I need to be. I know it is not his fault, but mine for hiding my emotions. Help me remember that tears are not a weakness but a gift you have given us to release these burdens that are so heavy. Help me to show our kids that it's okay to express themselves, good or bad, happy or sad so that they do not carry the pressure in their hearts or the pain in their shoulders that my family and I have done for several years. Free their spirits. Keep them safe and gleaming with your joy.*

I prayed and to journaled, waiting for answers. It seemed my emotions were taking over. The pain I felt inside became incredibly intense. Some days, I felt helpless. I began having nightmares of someone coming at me in my sleep. The dreams were very distressing. They were like shadows of demons attacking me.

JOURNAL ENTRY 5-17-08: *Dear God, thank you for today. Thank you for a great weekend, for the ability, the strength, the energy for all the activities with my kids. If feels so good to be active in their lives again. Thank you for time with my husband- help us to continue to grow in your love, to connect physically, mentally, emotionally, and spiritually. Keep him healthy and strong. Lord thank you for the message in the Narnia movie tonight, "Everything will come in its time". I don't know how to ask or what to do with this sensation behind my shoulder; it is so thick, so deep and so distressing to my chest, to my heart. Lord, I know you can heal all things. I trust you will heal this. I don't know if it is something that needs to be revealed, but I pray that you continue to take the fear of the unknown from me. I am sorry for my lack of faith sometimes. These dreams I have had were very upsetting but I know you are greater than anything, and that you will protect me always.*

JOURNAL ENTRY 5-19-08: *Dear God, thank you for today. It was a difficult day. Thank you for the resources I have to help me. This sign that my body is giving me is very scary because of its effect on my heart, the overwhelming emotion to cry and the fatigue it causes. Lord, thank you for giving me the strength and courage to ask for the help I need, and to share this with my husband. It's not easy for me. Thank you for healing me in so many ways. As I continue to heal please help it happen at the right place and the right time, when I have the support and resources I need. Please take the pressure in my chest, the overwhelming emotion, the skipped beats, the pain, all of it until it is time to be released, it's too overwhelming for me to handle without the support.*

Bring me to the right resource. This is making it very difficult to be a wife and mother right now. Help my kids and husband understand without worry or fear and let them know I am healing. Give me the time I need. Thank you, God. Jesus I love you. May your spirit be with me 24/7.

CHAPTER 14

Identity Crisis

I was so thankful for my resources. I cannot stress enough, if you are ill, or facing tough times, keep many resources available. These can be people, praying, journaling, a favorite quiet place, whatever it may be that brings you hope and peace. As for me, I was very fortunate to have met the people I had met throughout my healing journey, Lisa, who had been doing some neural biofeedback (brain retraining) with me had become a great friend and resource for me. She helped me identify a part of these emotions that were controlling me.

I never really understood the meaning of 'identity crisis' until I experienced it. I had gone through so many changes in my healing I was beginning to lose sight of who I was. The nightmares I was having were spiritual attacks in my time of weakness. Satan loves to attack us at our weakest moments. Remember, where God is there cannot be fear.

By identifying the fears, I felt much more at ease, and my nightmares stopped. I still felt the deep sensation of pain that was quite overpowering but I knew, as long as I kept my trust and faith in God, he would not show me anything I could not handle.

Dr. Prise helped me to see that there is great healing in facing our fears rather than avoiding them. It is true that if we face whatever is causing us to be fearful and allow God to show us, the outcome is always better than turning from it. When we turn from it, we may think it is easier to move forward, or that things are better left unknown, but the truth is that there are valid reasons behind our fears that keep us from being the person God created us to be and finding peace in our lives.

Fear is nothing more than being afraid of the unknown. The irony of fear is that if the things we are fearing took place, we would have what we needed to overcome it. The truth is that most things we fear never take place. Something you can do to try to overcome your fears is the following: First make a list of your fear or fears. Second, list what might happen if those fears would happen and third, list the benefits of what might happen if those fears come true. By making this list, we construct a record of fears through which we have already walked and seen his great faithfulness; thus, we lay hold of hope for our future. Finally, the consuming fearful thoughts are eliminated, lessening the chances of those things we dread coming upon us.

> JOURAL ENTRY 5-29-08: *Dear God, thank you for today. Thank you for the treatment with Micha. Please heal this mass, the pain, this annoying thing behind my right shoulder blade. Please take it, and let it be gone when I awaken. Give my body strength and stability where it is needed without any further injections or treatments. You said "ask and you shall receive"- Lord I am asking for your divine intervention- you are my greatest physician. Heal me as I sleep tonight, and may I wake and be healed physically, spiritually and emotionally, in every cell of my body. I love you Jesus and I will praise your name. I promise to use the gift you*

*have given me with great respect and never abuse myself
again- I ask, heal me by morning.*

As you can see, I was getting desperate to be healed from this pain in my shoulder that held this overwhelming emotion. Well, I was not healed by morning, but I did receive the strength to move forward and continue on my healing journey. During this time, I was gaining more energy and strength and really feeling anxious to return to work. It had been so hard to completely give up what I loved and felt so called to do. I knew it was not time yet. I knew I still had a lot of healing to walk through, and I did not have a peace about returning yet. I knew I owed it to myself and to my patients to wait.

It was June 13, 2008, and I received 119 prolotherapy injections in my thoracic spine and right shoulder. Dr. Weldon said it felt like I had tearing along the entire right scapula (shoulder blade). No wonder I had so much pain. These injections seemed to trigger a lot of my heart arrhythmias and angry feelings that I could not understand. I noticed I was feeling very tired again. I was taking on more responsibility as I regained my health, and it seemed my family was falling back into our old routine. My husband was working longer hours, and I was finding myself taking on too much. I prayed for strength to ask for help where I needed it, and to continue to find balance in our life. I felt guilty asking Doug to help more and not work so much, because I knew how much he had given up over the previous year trying to care for me. I felt like I was complaining, and I wanted so much to have the strength and energy to care for my family, but my body just could not handle it. In the meantime, life continued, and I became distracted with some health issues of my son. It seemed I did not have as much time to think about my healing and I thanked God for the strength and energy I had to care for my family. It seemed the more simple I tried to make our life, the more resistance I received from my husband and children. I began to feel like the outcast.

Throughout my healing, my eyes were opened to many changes that needed to be made in our eating habits, so I began changing the foods we ate to more raw fruits and vegetables and unprocessed foods, and preparing more healthy meals. Well, unfortunately, this new way of eating was not always as tasty as the old because of the salts and other toxic ingredients that were eliminated, which we become so accustomed to eating. I knew it was not going to be easy, but I felt there was great truth and peace in it, so I continued. They slowly accepted it, since I am the primary cook in the family. It's amazing how food changes our attitudes, affecting the decisions we make because of its altering chemicals in the brain. You can think of it as putting bad gas in a car. If we don't get the right fuel we don't run well, and everything starts to slowly breakdown. I began to see that suffering is sometimes needed to bring about discipline in our lives.

One thing I would highly suggest when you are ready to make changes to your diet and your family's diet is DO IT SLOWLY! I made the mistake of trying to make a change almost overnight. I have the discipline of doing whatever it takes to feel better and regain my health. When I learned of the toxins in the foods we were eating and the benefits of fresh and raw fruits and vegetables, it was hard for me to consume the usual boxed, canned items we were used to, much less feed them to my family so I made drastic changes. This was wrong, for a couple of reasons. First, you cannot expect everyone to have the same discipline, especially when they are not ill and do not understand the effects of toxic food, since they may not be experiencing any of the symptoms beyond what they think is "normal", especially children/teenagers. Second, such a drastic change can make a person ill. When we change from a toxic diet to a more healthy diet of raw fruits and vegetables, our bodies will naturally want to "clean house" and eliminate toxins of the liver; doing this too quickly can cause the liver to shut down. It is important to consult with a healthcare professional when making any significant dietary change.

We had also been trying to make a very important decision about home schooling. My son Lucas had asked me to home school, but honestly, I did not take him very serious, in the beginning. I thought there was no way I would ever be able to home school. My husband was not in favor of it at all. I began to pray about it, and I felt God guiding me toward home schooling, but I continued to try to resist it. I received a lot of negative comments from family and friends about home schooling. They had some concern that it would be too much for me to take on, due to my recent health issues.

No matter how much I tried to resist, it seemed God was showing me bold signs to make this shift in the schooling of our children. Even though my husband did not like the idea, he agreed to give it a try, and we made the decision to begin home schooling. I thank God that he made this change in our lives. By having the three youngest at home we began to realize that Lucas was having difficulty with reading. He had some struggles in school, but his teacher felt that he was having a problem with self-esteem. I did not agree with her, because of my five children, he was the most outgoing in all other areas. I began to realize Lucas' struggles with reading were causing him to be more withdrawn in school. After more attention and investigation, we discovered that his brain was not communicating with his eyes, which was causing him to see double as well as seeing letters backwards, a condition called exophoria. He could see with one eye, which is why we realized he would often tilt his head and cover one eye when trying to read. His eyes did not work together. We found out this condition was treatable, even reversible, at his age, so we began his treatments. I do not know that we would have discovered his struggle if we had not been homeschooling. I realized just how many children must go through school with a similar problem that keeps them in a group labeled 'slow' or 'learning disabled'. When I look back now, I see all the glory it has brought us, and I am so grateful God gave me the strength to recover and guided us to this decision. If I had not become ill and been forced to slow down, I may have missed out on this part of God's plan for our life, because I was too busy trying to fix everyone else and was not aware my family's needs right in front of me.

It is important to realize that we may be gifted in work outside the home and have good intentions; however, family is where our lives must begin. By caring for ourselves first, we can better care for our children. We teach them discipline by setting a good example. If we can give the gift of discipline to our children, they will carry on that gift, so they can do the will of God in their lives. This will change generations to come.

I wrote daily in my journal, slowly making changes in our lifestyle, attempting to make it simpler. It seemed that the harder I worked at simplifying our life, the more distant I was feeling from my family, especially my husband. Despite this emotional separation, I still experienced God's peace, and somehow, I knew we would be closer in the end. I did not realize just how busy our family had been, all going our separate ways. I was actively seeking God's guidance in my life. It seemed the better I felt and the more I tried to return to 'normal activity', the more my symptoms would return. This became my guide in knowing my limits. The more I attuned myself to my body, listening to my symptoms, the more I could control them. I wondered if I would ever get past this point and be able to return to work. I missed doing my job as a therapist so much. The time was coming when I would return, but first, the work in me had to be completed. I soon met Deborah Sweet, a practitioner who specialized in the Tara Approach. She was another vital resource in helping me to heal my nervous system.

CHAPTER 15

Re-Patterning My Nervous System

JOURNAL ENTRY 7-5-08: *'Dear God, thank you so much for today. Thank you for revealing another detrimental part of my healing. Thank you for Deborah Sweet and the gift you have given her to help bring me to this point in my healing; it's all coming together this morning. These symptoms are 'my friends'. As scary as they have been, they are the words of truth, the voice of truth coming through. I realized through my. session with Deborah that part of the fear I experience comes from my two near-death experiences- 1ˢᵗ at birth and 2ⁿᵈ of June 6ᵗʰ, 2007 when I had the injection in my neck/ shoulder, and also with the death of the twin I lost. The noise I hear in my head is the flat line monitor when my heart stopped beating first as an infant and second with the injection. I feel the tightness In my chest, the tremors, the dizziness, the pain.*

God created our central nervous system not only to remember our earliest moments, but also to re-pattern shocks and traumas that we experience throughout our lifetime. It is these shocks and traumas that pattern our lives. For instance, many people go through life angry and get upset at the smallest things and don't know why. Chances are this pattern started early in life, and may not even be yours but a generational pattern that was passed on. Sometimes it is a smell, a touch, or the sight of someone or something that triggers an old pattern of behavior. These patterns may cause chronic pain, digestion problems, loss of hearing, poor eyesight, dizziness, loss of balance, heart palpitations or arrhythmias, headaches, eating disorders, or numerous other symptoms that seem to never get resolved with traditional medicine. The beauty of the nervous system, like all other areas of the body, is that it is capable of healing, thanks to God's unique design. If you suffer from an illness that has been a mystery to the medical field and there seems to be no answers, this may be an area you want to explore. If the nervous system is out of balance, chances are it is affecting another area of your body. Sometimes the symptoms are minor and are ignored, as life carries on. Eventually, however, the body gets to a point of overload from stress, toxins, fatigue, or whatever it may be. There may come a point of reckoning, at which the symptoms become life-threatening, leading to chronic illness, disability, or even death. It is through becoming increasingly attuned to ourselves that we will find answers. Our bodies give us all the signs; all we have to do is "listen". Pray for God's guidance in leading you to the right resources, and He will take you there. Remember, "If God brings you to it, He will bring you through it". Sometimes our symptoms may bring us much fear and lead us to many expensive tests with no answers. However, if we can tune in and listen to what our body is telling us and face those fears, we will get real answers and healing. God did not intend for us to live a life of pain and illness. Our trials and sufferings help us grow, learn discipline, and be stronger disciples of Christ, if we trust and have faith.

The form of healing therapy to which I have referred here is called Jin Shin Tara. I have to admit, I was very skeptical in the beginning. However, when I finally began to take the self-care classes, which I was really doing for my patients, I began to become aware of sensations in my body that were very uncomfortable. They were reproduced and calmed. I found the self-care techniques to be crucial to my healing. I had tried all the traditional ways of medicine, but I was getting no relief or answers. As life-threatening as some of my symptoms felt, I began to refuse further medical testing and suggestions, since they just were not helping, and I was growing tired of the stress it was adding to my condition.

Although the Jin Shin Tara treatments seemed strange to me I felt a peace within me, which assured me this was the direction I needed to go. It was really out of my comfort zone, but the more I prayed about it, the more it seemed to be the right answer. There were family members that questioned what I was doing, telling me to be "careful", because of things they had heard about treatments like this. As a lifelong Christian, I was very careful to avoid anything that involved something that would direct me away from my faith. I really had a peace about it and felt God was trying to show me something, and I wanted to know what it was. I once shared this with my mother, and she remarked, "Well, sometimes things are better left alone". I thought that was a strange comment, but I did not really think much of it.

The more I went through treatments the more I was having memories of my childhood and questions of why I responded to situations the way I did. For instance, when I become upset about something, I shut down and try to alienate myself from others. I do not like others to see me upset, and I have a very difficult time sharing my feelings. For as long as I can remember I could not stand for anyone to put a hand on me or try to comfort me, especially my mother. I felt bad for acting that way toward my mother but something inside of me caused a great resistance toward her trying to get close to me. The feeling was like that of a child, who having just been hit by his mother, resists her subsequent attempts to reach out and hold him. Another example is my terror of needles. I could never understand why the sight of a needle bothered me so much that it would activate my nervous system, causing nausea and fainting. I could not remember a traumatic experience that would cause my body to respond that way. I soon found answers to these questions. I will explain in the next chapter.

I continued to pray each day for healing, pouring out my heart in my journal. It seemed that my focus was on strength and support to handle whatever came my way. I felt a very strong sense that I would need a lot of support. I did not know why, but the emotions surfacing in me seemed powerful and overwhelming. I noticed the Jin Shin Tara treatments that were surfacing my memories, which were connected to the thickness and pain I felt in my right shoulder. They were also re-activating my heart arrhythmias (skipped heart beats) and tachycardia (rapid heart rate). Although these sensations were uncomfortable and scary, I felt a peace that everything was going to be OK, and that God was allowing these memories in order to facilitate my healing.

I continued with the prolotherapy with Dr. Weldon. We decided injecting the right shoulder and wrist would help the instability and pain I had in that shoulder. This was an area I very much feared having injected. Not only because of the thought of more needles going in me, but also because it would involve shooting the front of my shoulder around the same site of the earlier injection, which caused my second near- death experience. I felt a great amount of respect and comfort with Dr. Weldon. She always started the injections with a prayer, and I knew she allowed God to guide her hands, so I would be safe.

JOURNAL ENTRY 7-24-08: *"Thank you for today, this was my fourth round of prolotherapy. It was very painful in my shoulder and wrist. Thank you for giving me the strength and courage to allow Dr. Weldon to inject the front of the shoulder/collar bone area. It was very scary facing the fear of what happened with Dr. H., when he injected there. Thank you for her prayers and her blessed hands. Help give me the rest I need. Help me to feel Doug's compassion and his love. I feel so empty with him sometimes, so distant. I need that connection with him. I don't want his pity. I just need to feel he cares. I need to feel the love in his heart and his hands. I want to make our marriage stronger every day. Thank you so much for the physical healing.'*

I felt the need for greater strength in our marriage. We have always had a good marriage, but there were times I needed Doug to have more compassion and to really listen to me. I felt so alone and empty sometimes, even with him right next to me. I didn't know how to explain it to him without causing an argument. He always meant well, and he was there for me anytime I asked, but he wanted to fix everything, and I just needed him to listen. Since I was not good at sharing my feelings, it was very hard for me to explain how I was feeling to him. As God says, "...Ask and you shall receive...". The more I asked for strength in our relationship, the more my prayers were answered. It was not very easy. We actually grew more distant for a while, but eventually we were led to a marriage encounter weekend that was the answer to our prayers and made our marriage better than ever. I will explain more in chapter 21.

I began having pain in my jaw and headaches again. I suffered from this pain as a young child and had not experienced it in at least 10 years, so I assumed it must be re-activation to allow healing. We often go through a re-activation of pain or symptoms when we do not allow something to heal right the first time. An example might be a child having chronic ear infections that are treated with antibiotics. These ear infections may show up later in life out of nowhere, not necessarily with the actual infection, but the body may feel the pain, because it was never allowed to heal right, due to the use of antibiotics. The memory has been stored in the tissue, waiting for a time we can 'listen' to it and correct what may have been the source of the pain. Other symptoms that began to happen to me included: increased heart rate, skipped beats, dizzy spells, tingling sensation in my legs, tightness in my chest, pain in the right side of my neck and jaw, headaches, irritability, irregular period with cramping and clotting, fatigue, thoracic pain, right wrist pain and a constant sensation of needing to stretch.

From what I had learned up to this point, these were many of the symptoms of nervous system shock, so I continued to pray and ask for God's guidance for answers.

JOURNAL ENTRY: 8-6-08: *'Dear God, please show me what these symptoms mean. Take my healing to the core level. Take me to the place and people that I need for this to happen. Give me the time for this healing. Help me to sleep well tonight. I love you, Jesus.'*

As I have already stated, "The closer you get to the core of an onion, the more it makes you cry". This is true with healing. It is those deeper layers at the emotional and spiritual level, which affect our central nervous system, that are the most difficult to work through. I am convinced these are the areas of chronic pain and disabilities some people live with that never seem to get resolved. These are the mysteries of healing that go unresolved in the medical world, because there is not a "typical" diagnostic test to name these ailments, and they do not make logical sense to the patient or physician. So the person continues to live with the pain and disability, or they get labeled as being a hypochondriac or having some type of mental illness. In the worst cases, death results, because of the body's inability to fight the overwhelming experience. God does not intend for us to live with pain, and there is always an answer. So it is important to have faith and never give up hope.

CHAPTER 16

The Core of My Healing

It is your faith that will bring you victory. Our attitudes will play a crucial role in our healing. Facing our emotional hurts and spiritual fears can be very difficult. Some people choose to face them which provides a healing experience beyond words. There is a peace that surpasses imagination at this level of healing. Others choose to continue on the road they are on, utilizing survival mechanisms to help them get through each day. Maybe it is not the right time in their life for this stage of healing, or it is just too overwhelming or fearful to face. If you are at this stage, just remember that with God there is no fear, and if he brought you to it, he will bring you through it. If you pray daily and trust, God will show you truth.

On my part, this was a time in my healing in which I chose to move forward, despite the fears I had. I felt pain so deep inside of me; I thought I would not be able to stop crying. The crazy part was that I did not know where the pain came from, or what it was about. I only knew that the more I prayed, the more I felt God guiding me to the answers. My prayer was that if there was something in my life that needed to be revealed, he would show me, and if I did not need to see the issue, that he would just take it from me. Deep inside, I wanted him to quietly take it, because I knew it was going to be very difficult to face. The feeling was like a mother losing a child, or a child losing their mother. My reluctance to face these things was reminiscent of Jesus praying in the Garden of Gethsemane, **Matthew 26: 39 "My Father, if it is possible, let this cup pass from me; yet, not as I will but as you will".** It seemed all I heard on K-LOVE that week was *"Whatever Your Doing"* by Sanctus Real. All I heard over and over again was a line that declared emphatically, *"It's time for letting go"*.

CHAPTER 17

Shocking Answers!!

It happened on the day of my neuro-endocrine continuing education class. I was anxious to take this class. I just knew it was going to give me answers to help our family's hereditary ailments, which we all had in common.

JOURNAL ENTRY: 8-9-08: Dear *God, thank you for today. Thank you for this beautiful day. Thank you for my life, for healing-for Micha, Stephanie, Margo, all those surrounding me and holding me up in prayer last night. Thank you for the time my husband is giving me. Help him to feel comforted that I am healing and doing well. Thank you for healing at the speed of light. Thank you for revealing the core of my pain and instability. You are an amazing God. Thank you for the strength you have allowed me this past year and the courage to move forward. Thank you for forgiveness I feel for my mother. Lord, please guide me in speaking to my parents, in the right time and place. Let me know if I should speak to them together or separate, now or later.*

Lord, allow this to heal generations past and generations forward. Thank you for using me as your healing vessel. Guide me through my continued healing, and show me when I am supposed to return to work. I have waited so long, as you know, and I am so hungry to do your work. Help me know when, where, who, how many-I want to do your will.

In a session during this class, I went through what is called a prenatal regression. This is simply a memory of a shock or trauma that happened prenatally. How can a person remember something before their own birth? It is not a conscious memory, but it rests at a subconscious level. It is a memory that was placed in our nervous system from the beginning. Remember, our nervous system is the first part of our being to form. All we experience from our conception throughout our life is stored in this amazing nervous system created by God. You can think of it like a computer's hard drive. Once information is placed in the memory it remains there. This information may be forgotten but it can always be retrieved unless the mother board (our brain) is destroyed (death occurs).

Anyway, as the class progressed throughout the day, I was feeling very uncomfortable. I began feeling very nauseated and had a headache that intensified as class went on. I began to feel the deep emotional pain I had been experiencing, and I could not stop the tears from flowing. It seemed all we talked about was stimulating my nervous system beyond my control. I kept trying to resist it, and I did not want others to see me in this state of mind.

Toward the end of the class, I was asked if I wanted to participate in a demonstration. My mind was telling me, "No, not in front of all these people!", but the rest of me was clearly ready and needed this treatment at this time. I agreed, and I felt a distinct peace about it, so I knew it was the right thing to do. As I climbed onto the table, Dr. Mines placed her hands over pulse points (not the pulse from blood flow but from the energetic pathways that run throughout our body). I immediately began to regress into a memory of myself in-utero during the first few months. This was clarified by the shape and size of the tiny fetus I was remembering. I could see myself hiding in a corner and I felt very cold. I was scared, but I had a bright light around me and felt God's presence around me in this womb. As Dr. Mines placed her hands on different pulse points and asked what I was feeling, the memories became clearer to me, and my headache intensified and I began to have severe tremors. I was trying to fight what I was remembering and did not think I could go on, but, with the support all around me, I was able to. I could see a large needle entering the uterus I was living in and I immediately got a horrible taste in my mouth (one I had experienced most of my life but did not know why) and then I began to vomit. I could not stop the reactions, I felt like I had been poisoned and my body was trying to eliminate it. It was at that point I realized that the injection given to my mother at that time (probably 4-6 weeks in-utero) nearly took my life.

This memory, which just bombarded me on that table, had allowed me to relive the experience, but even more than that, to re-pattern the shock that my nervous system had been holding on to all my life. It was very difficult for me to believe all I experienced during that session, but the peace I felt after this event was profound, and I knew at that moment that it had to be true and orchestrated by none other than God. I immediately felt such forgiveness for my mother, and I wanted to let her know. I began to see where much of my behavior came from throughout my life. I had always felt unwanted and out of place. Don't get me wrong. I was well taken care of and had a very loving family. It seemed all my life I would try my hardest to do anything that pleased others. No matter how much I was invited, I always had this feeling I was not really wanted. My mother would always say, "You may have been an unwanted pregnancy but you were not and unwanted child". Now I understood why she would go into such detail of how she was so tired, and that she had just been in the hospital to have her varicose veins stripped and was very surprised to find out she was pregnant with me right after her surgery. She seemed to carry such pain when telling about her pregnancy with me. She told me that when I was born I nearly died, because of a condition called hyaline membrane. My lungs were not quite developed and I could not breathe on my own. She said the doctor told her I may not make it through the night. It was at this pivotal moment she prayed to God, saying, "I didn't mean it, I will take care of her". During the regression, I had a memory of my mother trying to stop my delivery (tensing her muscles, so as to not let me out) and then I remembered as I was delivered I saw my father anxiously waiting to hold me first. I had no memory of my mother holding me after my birth. I had another memory during a regression seeing my mother lying there as if she was in shock with no acknowledgement of my existence. I remembered just looking at her and wondering why she didn't want to hold me. I will explain what I learned about this from my mother a little later in my story. This rejection at such an early time in my life shaped who I am today. As negative as that may sound, I mean it in a positive way. I learned at this young age that I needed to try hard and do everything the best I could to survive and for fear of further rejection. It was all so clear to me and made so much sense. The beauty of it all was that I was really getting to know the real me, and I could now move forward to be the person God created me to be, without continuing with my prenatal origin of behavior.

Please understand that I do not blame my mother in any way for the experience I had. It is part of who I am and I am very thankful that she had the strength to give me life. She has always had a strong faith about her, and, in the end, she trusted that God would give her what she needed to take care of me. She did care for me, and she continues to do so today. I am sure her suffering has been greater than mine in many ways. This whole experience has not only healed depths in me I could never have imagined but it has allowed my mother to be a great advocate for the pro-life movement.

CHAPTER 18

Rejection All Over Again

JOURNAL ENTRY 8-10-09: *Dear God, thank you for today. It has been a bit difficult. It is so hard to allow myself to heal as I need, and to be with my family. Please give me the time, without taking time from them. After my session the other night I felt so angry, but so many things in my life finally made sense. Then you came to me again throughout the night and healed layers in me, giving me forgiveness for my mother in my heart. I felt so free for the first time in my life. Then I spoke with my mother and she denied it mostly, or seemed not to be aware. I feel like she took the freedom I felt and brought me anger all over again. Lord, I know you were with me through all of this, and you still are. I don't know if the injection was known by my mother or unknown, or if it is too painful for her to have the awareness. I just know I need to move forward and know that whether she knows or not, whatever the truth may be, it will free generations back and generations forward. Please free me of this anger, Lord, and free my mother.*

> *Allow her to forgive herself. Help me to be able to share*
> *this with my husband; I need to, I want to, but I don't*
> *know that he will believe me or give me the support I*
> *need. He's not very good at comforting me in these times.*
> *I really need him. It's times like these I really need him,*
> *but I seem to push him further away. Help me to speak*
> *my needs and receive the support I need from him. Help*
> *me to sleep well again. The last two nights have been*
> *difficult. I love you.*

I was so confused. I began to wonder if everything I experienced was truth. I felt such a peace and forgiveness for my mother. For the first time in my life I truly felt the love a child should feel for her mother and wanted to hug her and tell her I love her. Like I said earlier, I never liked it when my mother tried to comfort me when I was upset. I kept all my feelings hidden from her and I would feel extremely agitated when she reached out to touch or hug me, and this always bothered me but I did not know why. I really needed confirmation from her that what I experienced was real, but instead, I felt rejection all over again. When I confronted her, she looked so confused, as if what I was telling her was not real. She even suggested, at one point, that perhaps I needed to talk to a priest. I felt so angry and confused. Maybe I was crazy. I began to regret confronting her about the whole situation, because the peace and forgiveness I felt was taken away once again.

Now my prayers seemed to focus more on support and understanding from my husband. I was not able to share this new awareness with him for several weeks and felt more anger and greater distance between us each day. I felt so alone. He was my best friend and I really needed to share this with him, but I was so scared of his reaction. I just knew he would think the whole thing was crazy and would not believe me, so I continued to keep it to myself. I prayed each night that God would bring us closer and help strengthen our marriage. I prayed for Doug's understanding of my feelings and for my strength and confidence to share my feelings with him. It's hard to believe we had been married for 16 years and known each other for 22 years, and still, I could not share my deepest feelings with him. Keeping it inside was tearing my heart apart. My symptoms of dizziness, fatigue, insomnia and heart arrhythmias seemed to have gotten worse.

Finally, after a couple of weeks, I was able to share my experience with Doug. I was having so much anger and so many crying episodes, he probably thought I was already crazy, and keeping it in only made my behavior worse toward him and the kids.

I felt a lot of relief sharing my experience with him, but, at the same time, I felt like I was trying to convince him it was all true and not just in my head. He was supportive and held me while I cried, but I had the sense he did not believe me, and he was not really hearing me. Obviously, I was feeling very frustrated and lonely. I could not get the empathy I usually was able to get from my mother, and I just did not feel like I was getting the emotional support I needed from my husband. I was so thankful to have my friends Micha and Margo. They really had a deep understanding of what I was experiencing, and they always had just the right prayers at just the right time. I continued to write my thoughts and cry out more than ever for my husband and me to find what we needed to bring us closer in every area. I needed his emotional support now more than ever. It seemed the more I tried to share with him, the more difficult our relationship became, and the more anger and frustration I felt, which only led to arguments. I felt like my whole world had been turned upside down.

JOURNAL ENTRY 9-10-08: *Dear God, please show me and Doug balance and peace in our lives. Show us where we are needed for your will. Bring us in union like you are with us. I love you Jesus.*

I continued to try to cope each day, but it was so difficult. There were times I wished I had never become aware of this experience. I continued to struggle with being around my mother, or even speaking to her. I felt very uncomfortable being near her and wondered if our relationship would ever be the same. She would not bring up our discussion, but she began complaining of pain and pressure in her chest, heart palpitations and difficulty sleeping. When I gave her physical therapy/cranial treatments, she would often tear up and bring up the fact that I was not an unwanted child but an unwanted pregnancy because of the timing in her life. She would often tell me how thankful she was that God gave me to her. I was able to tell her I forgave her no matter what happened, and I felt a great relief. On the other hand, I felt guilty for ever bringing up the experience, because I could see the distress it was causing in her. I did not want to resurface old wounds. It was confusing and difficult!

> JOURNAL ENTRY 9-19-08: *Dear God, thank you for today. Thank you for my session with Micha. Thank you for showing me to move forward and not backwards. Always remind me of Luke 1:45: "Blessed is she who believes what the Lord has told her." Please don't let these hard days discourage me. Help me continue to move forward. Show me if there is any reason not to return to work. Please show me where I belong, who I am. I am looking forward to this retreat tomorrow (I had a retreat planned for caregivers). Show me what I need, lift my spirits. May there be great healing this weekend. Thank you for my time with Raeley (my daughter) today. She has a great spirit.*

I tried to return to work at this point, but it did not take me long to realize, through prayer and noticing the symptoms in my body, that it was not time yet. As much as I wanted to return,

I knew I had more healing to receive in myself first, before I could help others. I was still experiencing a lot of pain in my hip and back. This time, I chose to listen to my body, and I did not continue to work.

CHAPTER 19

Marriage Encounter Weekend

Doug and I continued to struggle in our relationship. It was still difficult for me to share my deepest feelings. I continued to pray for our guidance and strength in our marriage. Ask and you shall receive! My prayers were answered. By October we made it to a World Wide Marriage Encounter Weekend. We had been told about them in the past and always wanted to attend one, but it never worked out, until now. God knew it was the right time, and we needed it now more than ever. Although we had a good marriage, it seemed our ability to communicate had gotten worse over the past few years. It seemed that the more I walked through my healing, the more I needed him. However, we grew increasingly further apart. Daily, I was becoming more frustrated and angry with him for not understanding my needs and not supporting me emotionally when I really needed him. I knew we had a strong foundation with God in our lives, so no matter how distant it seemed we were getting, I felt a peace that God was going to show us something, and that our marriage would be better than ever. It was only by God's grace that I held on to this faith because, at this time, we were barely speaking to each other anymore without arguing. As we progressed through the weekend, we began learning about tools to use through dialogue to improve our communication. By the second day, it was as if all the lights came on, and for the first time in 22 years, I felt like my husband finally listened and understood what I needed. I thanked God, as I cried tears of joy.

I knew this was a new beginning for us. I realized that I was doing a poor job of expressing my feelings to Doug, because I never really knew how. I realized that he was not insensitive but frustrated, because he could not "fix" my problems. He learned that all I needed was for him to support me by listening, and I did not want him to "fix" anything. I just needed him to understand how I was feeling. It seemed 99% of the couples in our class had the same issues. It was truly amazing to be a part of this encounter. I realized just how sacred marriage is. I never grasped the true meaning of the sacrament of marriage until we attended this weekend. I felt so ashamed that I had been so selfish about our marriage. I was always looking for ways to improve my relationship with my husband, but I had completely missed the fact that our marriage was a gift from God, and that we are to choose to love one another, for God, not ourselves. I learned that our marriage represents a small church within the church and that we are to choose to be an example of Christ's love by choosing to love one another, no matter what the circumstance. This is not always easy, but if we can remember the importance of our sacrament and live out our covenant, we will influence others to do the same. If you ever have a chance to attend a "World Wide Marriage Encounter" weekend, do it! Your marriage will never be the same. You will have a bond in your union, which nothing can break apart. Just google WWME, (World Wide Marriage Encounter) and you will find all the information you need. You can also ask about it in your church. Although it was formed through the Catholic Church, all are welcome.

From this point on, my pain became easier to live with. Nothing had changed physically, but now that I had my best friend, my husband, to share what I was feeling. Knowing he really understood made it easier emotionally to get through each day, I found a greater strength to deal with it each day and a greater hope to find healing, now that I had someone by my side who truly understood what I was feeling. I found myself pulling him closer and asking for help when I needed it, instead of becoming angry and pushing him away.

Together, my husband and I continued to search for answers to my heart arrhythmias and back/hip pain and instability. We met a new surgeon that was doing SI (sacroiliac) joint fusions. It seemed like an option for me for the first time in a long time, since this seemed to be where my pain and instability was centered, but we were not totally convinced this was my answer. In many ways, I wanted to have it done, hoping it would be just what I needed, but there was something telling me it may not be right, so I continued to research and pray about it. It seemed the more I prayed, the more roadblocks there were to getting this procedure done. The doctor seemed worried that I was still of child-bearing age, and that, if we chose to have this done, having another child would mean I would have to have a C-section. Although we had no plans to have more children, this really disturbed me. We chose to wait and continue to pray for an answer. One night, I asked God to bring me an answer in my dreams. That same night I had a dream that I was having an x-ray done, and there was a baby stuck in my pelvis. As I thought about this, I interpreted this to mean that God was not going to give us any more children because of my health, but that he was going to give me new life and healing in my back and hip. Boy, was I wrong about him giving us more children!

CHAPTER 20

Apls-Another Answer

In the meantime, I had consulted with Dr. Weldon about the idea of the SI fusion, and she strongly encouraged me not to have it done, and she asked to re-evaluate me before I made the decision, to determine if anymore prolotherapy would help. I decided to consult with her and Dr. Merriman, and they recommended I have a stronger solution injected into the SI joint without anesthesia, because the joint was still very unstable. I chose to have this done and it seemed to give me more stability. I decided to give the prolototherapy more time and put off the SI fusion.

JOURNAL ENTRY 11-27-08: *Dear God, thank you for answers. It is Thanksgiving morning. I am so grateful that you love me so much. The last several days I have felt the need for prayer from 2 or more. I keep hearing the verse- "where 2 or more are gathered in my name, there I will be". I sent an email to Micha last Friday requesting prayer with her and Margo. Again on Wednesday, as Gina was treating me in physical therapy, Ashley was observing and Pauline and Mary* came in the room. I wanted to ask them to pray for me but did not have the courage. One evening, as my husband was lying with me and talking to me, I wanted to ask him to pray for me, but again, I did not have the courage to ask him. I received an email the following Tuesday from Micha saying she and Margo would call and pray with me. It just so happened I did not have class that evening, and they prayed with me. I felt your presence God. The words 'courage and stability' seemed to scream at me as Micha prayed. My prayer was for 2 answers; my heart problem and my hip/back. I woke up early the next morning and could not go back to sleep. Your answers were flowing through me. My mom called me later that day telling me of a genetic disorder she had on her side of the family called APLS. She was not sure what it was, but she happened to have just talked to her sister and found out her sister's daughter had it. She had many of the same symptoms as me. It seemed to fit all my heart symptoms and many other things I had struggled with for years. So many answers are rushing in. Thank you, God. I hear your message being - courage is needed to stand up in your name Lord without hesitancy. Stability is needed in my hip. I saw your hands holding my hip in the socket as Micha prayed. I had been taping my back and hip for a couple years to give it stability. As I got up to journal, I grabbed the wrong notebook and came across old journals and notes that confirmed the APLS symptoms. I kept hearing a new song on K-love called - "Bring Me a Revelation"- it spoke volumes to me. Lord you have shown me this, guide me to the right doctor to diagnose and treat it. Guide me to the right doctor for my hip.

APLS is Antiphospholipid Syndrome which your immune system makes the mistake of making antibodies against certain proteins in your blood which can cause blood clots in the arteries or veins. I began to search for a doctor, who was familiar with this APLS disorder, but I found it was very hard to diagnose. I had difficulty finding a doctor that could test me for it. I was very frustrated, but I refused to give up, because I felt God had led me to an answer I needed to follow. About a month went by. Still, no answers. I began to get angry at God wondering why it was so difficult to get answers to what he had shown me. It was December, and I had a follow up appointment with Dr. Weldon for the prolototherapy. I had a bad feeling about any further injections she was going to do around the neck and shoulder for my shoulder pain and thoracic outlet syndrome, which she felt was contributing to my heart arrhythmias. I explained to her what I had learned about the possibility of having APLS. She was very concerned, and she told me she could have me tested for it.

> JOURNAL ENTRY 12-10-08: *Thank you for today. Thank you for this trip to Tulsa and my time with Dr. Weldon. Thank you for insight and protecting me from the trauma that may have resulted from a blood clot. Guide Dr. Weldon to order the right tests, so that I may have answers for the right treatment. Guide me to the right treatment for my hip. Thank you for more answers. My hip arthro-gram that I asked Dr. Robbins to order has revealed my instability. Finally! After 20 years of back and hip pain and instability, the arthro-gram showed that I had a detached anterior labrum (the tissue that holds the hip in the front of the socket) and a torn iliofemoral ligament (the ligament that attaches the hip to the leg). Thank you, Lord, for more answers.*

Knowing this, the SI fusion would have been a disaster. If I had gone through with the surgery for the SI fusion, my pain and instability would have been so much worse. Also, with the possibility of having APLS, I was at great risk of throwing a blood clot which could have taken my life. Dr. Weldon confirmed that, if I had APLS, she had no doubt that what I experienced after the inter-scalene injection. was several mini-strokes.

A few weeks later it was confirmed. I did have APLS. I immediately started taking aspirin daily to thin my blood. I noticed a difference fairly quickly. I had some increased energy and less foggy headedness. I was only taking 81mg a day and felt I needed more, but I did not want to overdo it, so I stuck with the 81mg. It all happened in the right time. We had planned a ski trip to Colorado a few days after Christmas. I cannot imagine what it would have been like in the mountains if I had not started on the aspirin. I noticed increased symptoms of fatigue and foggy headedness while we were there so I took extra aspirin, which helped. Later through blood tests I found my blood was so thick I needed 325 mg daily. Dr. Mines describes the developmental stages as blood circulation being established in prenatal development at week 4 in utero. She also notes, "the head and tail are formed which means there is brain and spinal cord development. Neural folds fuse and heart tubes fuse at midline. This is where the optic vessels appear, nostrils appear, and the beginning of the lungs, liver, stomach, pancreas, and thyroid. The upper limb buds appear, leg buds appear, heart development increases, and the optic lens forms." As you can see this is a crucial part of development, which is happening typically before the mother even knows she is pregnant or has just become aware of her pregnancy and where many abortions take place. Becoming aware of the shock in my prenatal regression is a crucial part of healing my heart. Every time I went to a heart doctor my best explanation was that "I felt like I was being shocked or that I had a short circuit in my heart. I felt like someone would turn off the main breaker in me that controlled my electrical system and everything would shut down and I would proceed to blackout". Most of the doctors looked at me with confusion or like I was crazy. As I stated earlier, one diagnosed me with 'neurocardiogenic syncope', which he described as a nerve somewhere in the body causing this to happen, but they did not know why and there fix to be an ablation (burning of the artery) or a pacemaker. It is an answer and a temporary fix for many but God has given me strength to seek out the truth.

> JOURNAL ENTRY 12-25-09: *Happy Birthday, Jesus. Thank you for this day Lord. Thank you for allowing me to share this awesome day with you, family and friends. Thank you for our health. Thank you so much for family. Lord, help continue to guide each and every one of us to your will. I look forward to the New Year. Thank you for who I am, for showing me who I am. Help me continue to be grateful each and every day no matter what. Let your light shine through me. I praise you, Lord. Thank you for this joy you give me. Help my brain continue to heal and my hip, back and shoulder- my body as a whole. Continue to guide me to the right resources. Keep me from any unnecessary appointments. Keep our family safe on our way and back from Colorado. Keep our family safe who are meeting us there. I give thanks for this vacation. I give it to you, Lord. Help me sleep well tonight. I love you, Jesus.*

We returned home safely. I searched for answers for my heart symptoms and shoulder pain. Many days, I felt very overwhelmed trying to heal and care for my children at the same time. I was taking the aspirin, as well as another natural blood thinner. It all seemed to help, but I continued to have irregular heart rhythm and dizziness. I knew there were more answers I had to keep searching for.

> JOURNAL ENTRY: 1-14-09: *Dear God, thank you for today. I have not slept well the last couple nights. It seems we have been so busy my brain can't stop. Lord, help us to slow down. Show me my limits. Help me to be where you want me. Thank you for the healing. Continue to guide me to the right resources. I am so thankful for the strength to care for my kids, but I feel so overwhelmed some days. Please give me the strength, the energy, the help I need with them and caring for my family. Guide us in the right help for Lucas and his learning and vision difficulties. Show us truth in it all. Help me to have the time I need for my book, and help me take one day at a time and not rush my healing. Please help me find answers to this mass behind my shoulder- it is so difficult living with the pain and neurological, sympathetic (increased heart rate, heart arrhythmias) symptoms it causes. I pray the prolotherapy will heal it 100%. In my session with Micha the other day, she mentioned "spiritual strangulation"??? If there is something you need to show me Lord, something that is strangling my spirit, set it free- show me what I need. I trust you Lord and I want to be free from anything that keeps my spirit anxious or fearful, anything that keep me from complete peace. I love you, Jesus.*

I learned nearly two years later what the 'spiritual strangulation' was about. I will explain in Chapter 24.

The more I paid attention to the pain in my shoulder, the more anxiety I felt when it flared up. It had a pain and numbness, which, to me, was so deep, I could not reach it. I could not relieve it, no matter what I tried. I would often have someone stick their elbow on my shoulder and push as hard as they could, but I could never get them to push hard enough. Nothing relieved the pain.

As I prayed and searched for answers I received more answers in a dream one night. This dream told me my heart problem was electrical, but I did not need a pacemaker, and Stephanie could help. Stephanie was the doctor, who practiced Jin Shin Tara. The electrical part that was affecting my heart was causing actual physical symptoms, not because of a heart defect, but because of electrical imbalance of the cells from past shocks and traumas I had experienced. She had helped me in the past with my awareness of the shocks and traumas of my prenatal life, by re-patterning my central nervous system. Through this dream, I had a peace that I would find answers. The fears and anxieties concerning my symptoms seemed to lessen. I knew God would guide me to more answers. I continued to remind myself to be grateful for each day, in spite the symptoms I was still experiencing.

> JOURNAL ENTRY 1-29-09: *Dear God, thank you for today. Thank you for the success of my prolotherapy (144 injections to the cervical spine and ribs, 16 injections to L4-5, and an HGH injection to the right hip). I am in a lot of pain, but your peace is upon me, and the healing has begun. Thank you for the help and support of my husband. Thank you for the calmness of my heart. Thank you for revealing the aspirin I need to take, 325mg instead of 81mg. That sense I needed of taking more was right. Help me to believe in myself, to have self-worth, to act on your truth when I feel it. I am so grateful for your Holy Spirit to guide me. Thank you for the rest I am getting. Thank you for our wonderful kids. Help me to sleep well tonight. Help Doug and I make the right decision about our insurance. Show us truth; give us faith to leave it in*

your hands. Take any selfishness or attitude that keeps
us from your truth. I love you, Jesus.

I received more prolotherapy along with the use of the aspirin. Dr. Weldon's prayers before my treatments eased my fears of all the injections that were involved. I felt that this would help the pain and weakness in my arm and in the thoracic outlet, which contributed to my heart arrhythmias. Deep down, however, I knew there was more to this healing journey. I still had a deep pain, along with a sense of numbness in my shoulder, which was connected to my heart arrhythmias and also to a feeling of disconnection from Doug. I knew this was so, but I could not understand why. I prayed and journaled for answers.

This brought me to my next session of Jin Shin Tara with Stephanie. During this session, I had an awareness of me and my father when I was about 2 or 3 years old. There was such a sadness, which I soon could not stand to feel anymore. This awareness and the pain in my right shoulder were closely connected. I began to understand where part of my hormone imbalance came from. This imbalance affected my ligaments and my ability to feel sensations throughout my body. The points of imbalance in my nervous system affected the heart and pelvis, which contributed to decreased circulation, blood clots, and bladder and kidney problems. Somehow, these areas, afflicted at such a young age, were contributing to my physical ailments.

However, the sadness I felt in my heart was too great to move forward, at this time. I decided to continue with the self-care treatments of rebalancing my nervous system and follow-up with Stephanie next month, in order to find more answers. Now was just not the right time. After this session, I began to have more outbursts of anger, and I did not know where they came from. I hated this anger I felt inside of me, and I hated the person it caused me to be toward my husband and kids. I was having more skipped beats, and they were always distressing. At times, I felt so out of control, and the anger toward my husband seemed without cause or reason.

In the meantime, there was a lot going on. I had completed my year-long class of nutritional counseling. I continued to try to find time to complete my book and earn my Doctorate of Naturopathy. I was so thankful for the strength and courage God had given me to travel back and forth to Tulsa each week for a year, despite my struggles. I am grateful for the knowledge I gained through both that class and my own experiences. I looked forward to the day God would allow me to use all of it to help others. There were many times I was desperate to return to work and tempted to do so, but I knew God would show me when the time was right. I knew I had to focus on what he was healing in me before I could return. I had made that mistake in the past, and I was not going to do it again. It had been a hard lesson learned, but I realized I could not help others until I first helped myself.

> JOURNAL ENTRY 2-25-09: *Dear God, thank you for this day. Thank you for my time in the office, my treatment with Micha and Ashley. Thank you for the healing in my shoulder. Thank you for the beautiful message while listening to my CD of the rosary today. I ask of you, like Jesus did, if my cup runs over, please take it from me but let it be your will, not mine. I feel such a deep emotional pain in the right shoulder that is sometimes physically unbearable. Somehow, I know it is connected to my father. If this is not mine to carry, Lord, allow me to let it go. If there is something I need to know, give me strength and courage to see your truth. Protect me from confusion. Calm my heart, allow me to sleep well and rest in you, Lord.*

A week later, I received more prolotherapy (114 injections in my right hip and my second HGH injection in my right hip).

I knew this would be a great part of my physical healing. I wondered how I had managed to walk all these years. I was so grateful for the resources God had guided me to.

> JOURNAL ENTRY: 3-5-09: *Dear God, thank you for this day. I am getting a little nervous. My period is five days late. I am sorry for feeling this way. I would welcome the gift of a child, but it seems so unbelievable to imagine having another. I am still slowly healing. I feel I need more healing, and I feel too tired to have another. I know you will not give us more than we can handle, and I trust you. Let it be your will, Lord, not mine. Whatever that may be, give me strength. My son Lucas said to me today, "God told me something, but I can't tell you for six days". He has such a gift for hearing you, Lord. I practically knew, at this point, I was pregnant. After all, Lucas had told me I was pregnant with his last brother before I ever knew.*

We soon found out we were blessed with another child. As difficult as it seemed it would be, I felt a peace within that God would carry us through. I had a sense that, even though I struggled physically, somehow, this baby was going to bring me a lot of healing. It is often through having children that we are healed from our own shocks and traumas. This would prove to be the case with this pregnancy. It felt as though I was receiving some of the same feelings my mother had when she was pregnant with me. I was so grateful for the tools I had acquired to prevent prenatal obstacles that could have developed. With these tools I could not only stop negative generational patterning, but heal generations past including my other five children that may have received what I had carried my whole life. By sharing my experience with them or merely changing my behavior the generational patterning would be reversed and stopped.

JOURNAL ENTRY 3-23-09: *Dear God, thank you for this day. It has been a little difficult. I don't seem to be sleeping as well. My heart doesn't beat right, I am so tired and having some depression. I also notice some anger coming up again. This class I recently attended (Healing at the Speed of Light- combining manual therapy with energy medicine and balancing the nervous system) seems to be re-activating some things. I get very confused. With this awareness of my mother, I feel like it could bring us closer but her reactions seem to make it more difficult. I am not sure what to do with that, Lord. I am sad for her, but I know I cannot take her pain. I ask that you take anything that is not mine, concerning my family, and give it back to them. Help me to take what I have seen as truth and move forward in your light, continuing to become the person you created me to be. Help me to rely on your strength. Show me what you want me to see through this anger and sadness. Show me where you want me. Use me as a tool and allow your light to shine through me. I want to glow with your light, so others will see the peace you can bring, the truth. Guide me in my new wellness clinic. Bring me anyone you want me to serve. Provide what is needed. Let me rest in you Lord.*

Overall, my pregnancy was going well. Some days, I struggled with fatigue, but my energy was pretty good, considering I had 5 other children to take care of, I was home schooling, and I still had a business to manage, even though I was not physically working. I am so grateful for the wonderful husband I have, for his help in balancing our life, and for taking such good care of us. I continued to struggle with the heart arrhythmias on a daily basis, and I knew there were more answers for me yet to come. Sometimes, I still experienced agitation and a deep sadness that seemed to come out of nowhere. Instead of letting the anger and sadness control me, I began to try to pay attention to it, so I could learn where it was coming from, and how I could heal from it. The sadness seemed to have a significant connection to my father, which aggravated my heart arrhythmias. I did not understand what that connection was, but I knew God would show me in time. That week my oldest son, Caleb, whom has a great faith and trust in the Lord brought me a small stone that he bought me that said "let go, let God".

I also began to have strong urges to return to work again. Working as a manual physical therapist is not a job for me. It has become part of who I am, and it fills a part of me that brings me peace and joy. When I put my hands on someone, they seem to know where to go without my having to think about it. It's when I try to think about techniques that I struggle. If I just 'let go and let God', my hands are guided where they need to be, and I am able to be an instrument of God's work. I was very anxious to begin the wellness center and use all I had experienced and learned in the past year of study to help others.

I struggled with the decision to return to work, fearing I would overdo it and end up ill again. I was very frustrated that God had given me such a gift and I was not able to use it. I chose to take time to pray about my decision and return only when I felt a peace that God was calling me to do so.

> JOURNAL ENTRY: 3-30-09: *Dear God, thank you for today. I had a pretty good day. It started a little slow, but I thank you for the energy I got later. I feel I am being called back to treating patients in so many areas, but the pain and arrhythmias confuse me. Lord, I want to listen to my body and respect it this time, but at the same time, I am fearful and anxious to overdo it, and I feel this keeps me from treating and returning. I want to do your will, Lord, so if back to work is where you*

want me, and treating manually, then I ask you to let it happen, and do not let fear stop me from doing your will. Be my strength so that no energy or physical ailments break me. I am strong in you Lord- fill my spirit/my soul with great strength. Also, I often feel overwhelmed with home schooling but it feels so right. I know I can't do it all. Bring me the help I need. Allow me to ask for help. I love you, Jesus.

CHAPTER 21

Back to My Passion

One day, I decided to see a few patients, in order to help out, since we were booked, and the other therapists did not have any openings. It felt so good in many ways, but overall, I knew it did not feel right yet. When I treated, I still struggled with pain and with balance at home. I felt called to work as a therapist, but I knew my role as a wife and mother was priority. My husband did help with the kids, but I needed so much more help with the cooking, the cleaning, the home schooling. I felt guilty asking for more help from him, because he worked so hard outside of the home, but I knew I could not return to work outside the home without his support.

I received my last set of prolotherapy injections on April 7, 2009.which included HGH to the right hip and lumbar area, and some in the lower cervical and first rib area, which seemed to really affect my heart symptoms. Since I was a few months pregnant, I was not able to get anymore prolotherapy because my body would soon be affected by ligament laxity for the baby's growth, which would defeat the purpose of the injections to tighten the ligaments. This hip injection caused increased tremors throughout my body and triggered the sad feeling I experience when I am intimate with my husband. I am aware that emotion tied to hip pain often has to do with relationships, so I knew the feeling I was having must be connected to a memory.

I prayed that God show me what it was or take it from me, so I could move forward in my healing. I kept hearing the song *"Here I Am"* by Down Here. I heard the words in the song loud and clear that said, "I know you will finish what you began." Again, God was giving me messages of hope through the music I listened to. I continued to take one day at a time, trying to balance home and work. I struggled with loss of sleep and waking with night sweats, and I knew I needed to face these feelings I was having, so I could go on from this place. I was worried that the lack of sleep and heart arrhythmias were causing stress on the baby. I decided to schedule a therapy session with Micha and Margo. I felt very safe with them because of their spiritual strength, and I knew God would only reveal what he wanted me to know.

JOURNAL ENTRY 5-6-09: *Dear God, thank you for today. Thank you for my session with Micha and Margo. Help me to let go and move forward. You showed me today that whatever this emotional pain is when I was 2-3 years old is too much for me to handle right now, and that you will keep it for me until I am ready. Help me to trust in what I experienced today, Lord. Help me to move forward and not be curious about what you obviously don't need me to see. Help me to trust, to let go, and move forward. Take this memory until you are ready for me to see it. Thank you for the ability to forgive my mother. Help me to let go of the pain I see in my family and give it to you. Allow me to help only where I am needed, in your ways and not mine. Take the rest. I don't know where these headaches and jaw pain come from but please take them. Take this anger from me. Help me continue to find peace. I love you!*

We may not always get the answer we are asking for, but God does answer. Like the song says by Garth Brooks: "Some of God's Greatest Gifts are Unanswered Prayers". Again, He brought me what I needed. Again, ask and you shall receive! I did return to work a few more times before I was ready and God kept showing me that it was not time yet so I had to stop. I was almost embarrassed with the many times I returned and stopped because many patients who truly cared for my well being would question if I was really ready to return. I would look them straight in the eye and say, "yes I am ready or I would not be here". Then within a few weeks I would have to lay my pride aside and admit once again I was not ready. Obviously even my patients could see I was still healing.

CHAPTER 22

A Mystery Revealed

Journal Entry 4-8-10: Dear Lord, Wow!!! Thank you for the treatment. What a transformation. I think I grew 2 inches on the right side. You are healing my deepest structural deformities. My tissue has been shortened since birth due to trauma of my extraordinary meridians. The rotational (scoliosis) component is being freed. You have delivered me from this oppression. "My help comes from the Lord", and "The healing hands of God"; You have played these songs loudly over and over giving me the message that you would be the one to heal me. Although there were many reasons (TMJ dysfunction, no posterior communicating artery in my brain, a hole in my heart, scoliosis, many bulging and herniated discs, a fracture of my vertebrae, a right shoulder fracture, scar tissue of the organs, right hip dysplasia, anxiety and depression of unknow origin, chronic insomnia, nerve compression, auto-immune disease, etc.) you are healing it all. As I boldy and confidently speak of your healing, my breath expands. I am lengthened. Your light bursts through each cell. I am radiant with your light. Ask and you shall receive! With your strength, your grace, your perseverance, you are answering all my prayers. You have shown me I will do great things in your name. I love you Father, Creator of Heaven and Earth. **Revelations 2:3; "And you have perseverance and have endured for my name's sake, and have not grown weary."**

As I read over my journals through the next several months I noticed I kept asking for answers for my shoulder pain and the skipped heart beats I had felt for the past few years, especially while lying on my right side. This was a mystery no one could answer. I did find it odd that sometimes it would happen very often and then there were nights I could lay on my side and 'nothing!' I kept having the sense to finish my book before returning to work, but of course, I did not listen. Again, this was a great distraction for me not to finish. I realized that this was my answer. The answer the Lord had shown me over and over again. He had given me the strength and the words all along in preparation for this book. Now I had in mind that it was being written for my healing and really did not intend to share it. Well this obviously was not in God's plan. He has shown me over and over again, no matter how difficult, that he wants me to share it. This is part of his will for my life, an assignment he has given me that I have been reluctant to complete. You may wonder, what does this have to do with my symptoms and lying on my right side? It has been said, the emotional pain we carry on our left side is typically something from our past or from generational passing from one side of the family. Emotional pain carried on the right side typically deals with the present or from family.

I had been avoiding the completion of this book because I feared the outcome that it may bring, and of the vulnerability of my life experiences. First, I thought it would never be good enough to really let someone read it. Second, I feared having to live through the rejection I may get from family and friends. Finally, I found myself still doubting that what I experienced was real. This resulted in the unknown anger I kept feeling, which was ultimately anger toward my mother for not confirming this for me. Through much prayer I have found that the only thing not of truth was the doubt I was having. As I was explaining the importance of forgiveness to my daughter one evening I became aware that I had been holding on to the anger I had held in since my regression nearly 3 years earlier. I still had not received the confirmation I needed from my mother because of my own doubt of what God had shown me as truth. This was the "spiritual strangulation" Micha had talked about that she heard from the Lord nearly two years prior during one of my treatment sessions. I was stuck! As a friend/healthcare provider told me, our bodies are like a garbage disposal. If we hold on to the garbage in our life, whether it be ours or what belongs to others, we cannot progress. I found this to be affecting me physically more than anything. I noticed fatigue returning that was so debilitating, some days it took all I had to get out of bed. The nausea was so awful I was going several days with very little to eat, hence, making me sick to my stomach to keep it in. These were all symptoms I had continued to experience throughout my healing, but the difference this time was I felt strong underneath it all. I had built a strong foundation and was ready to heal from the core of my illness. By holding this information in I was causing toxins to hold in my tissues which were greatly affecting my liver and gallbladder. My digestion was struggling (even though I ate very well and exercised) so I could not release the toxins that had been stored, especially the heavy metals.

March of 2011 I received a treatment from my friend Kristi who is also a gifted healer and physical therapist and has a great gift to hear the Lord. During the treatment tears drenched my face as I was brought back to the memory once again of my birth. She gave me the words I needed to separate myself from my mother's wounds. I realized I was still carrying emotional shocks and traumas that did not belong to me. Through prayer and journaling, I was finally able to let go of what was not mine and stand on my own truth to fulfill God's promise. He has shown me since conception that He will protect me and there is nothing to fear. This led me to a fast, which completed the physical healing of my gallbladder. Through the fast I released several gallstones. How ironic that the first doctor I saw during my illness suspected I had a bad gallbladder. Deep down I felt she was right but I did not feel my answer was to have it removed. I have no doubt that if it had been removed, it would have been diseased with little to no function. Sure it may have given me temporary relief of my physical pain and heart symptoms but I may never have received the fullness of God's peace emotionally and spiritually if I had not listened to what God was showing me. The gallbladder is where we hold anger. Behind anger most often there is fear. This in turn affects our digestive system, which in turn affects our body as a whole, physically, emotionally, and spiritually. This may keep us from being who God created us to be.

I am guided by God through a song on K-LOVE; "My Help Comes from the Lord" by The Museum. As I journal each day and search, I am guided to the truth.

I have been led to many sources of help throughout my healing journey. There has been a multitude of resources that were a part of this amazing walk of faith, but my ultimate resource has been God himself. It is only when I learned to trust him and not myself that I was led down the right path, medical or non-medical. All along, I have been looking for the one day of breakthrough, when I would finally and forever be cured. However, I have learned I will be healing throughout my lifetime here on earth, whether it is physically, emotionally, or spiritually. I have learned what it means to fear the Lord and to lean on Him when the deceptions of this world creep into my life. Our ultimate healing comes from the Lord, and if we listen, He will guide us to good health and peace on earth, as it is in heaven. There may be obstacles along the way, but are these obstacles what brings us the health God has promised us? It is our perseverance, through God's grace, that allows us to overcome them.

CHAPTER 23

Logic or Truth

My story of healing continues, and God is still revealing answers. I look forward to sharing these answers and what God has in store for me in my next book. He has shown me that by completing this book I have completed one of many assignments. Even greater, by sharing this book it will allow me to be the person He created me to be as well as bring answers to others in search of healing.

I finally chose to obey the Lord and share the rough draft of my book with my parents and received the confirmation as of all my prenatal experiences as God had promised. In many talks with my mother and father they were able to confirm that several of the memories I had had through my regressions were true, even the memory of my father being the first to hold me. My mother shared that she does not remember holding me after birth until the next day when the doctor delivered the news that I may not survive. She cannot remember why she did not hold me; she feels it may be due to the harsh anesthesia they used back then. She did share with me for the first time, that she had asked God to take me from her because she did not feel she had the strength to care for another child.

I had been confused, wondering if my mother had actually tried to abort me. Between my memory of the injection and the timing of her surgery I was convinced that what I experienced was not and could not possibly be an attempted abortion. It had never made sense to me because of my mother's strong beliefs against abortion. By to share sharing this book with my parents, God cleared up part of this confusion. Instead of holding on to what God showed me I began to search for what logically made sense. I had convinced myself that what I experienced was actually what is called "Annihilation Ideation" as defined by Dr. Mines. According to her definition in her book, **Pre and Perinatal Psychology**, this event is "one of the most severe forms of shock". She defines annihilation ideation as "feeling a projected desire for the death of a child developing in utero". The key feeling felt by a child who experiences this can be one of always feeling their life is in danger or always feeling they have to be on guard. Symptoms of abortion survivors may include struggling to claim one's existence, depression to the point of suicide or self-destructive behavior. They may also experience a feeling of being suffocated or dominated by other people's needs, which can physically result in asthma or respiratory illness. Abortion survivors can have compromised autoimmune function. Dr. Christiane Northrup provides validation for this statement through a number of scientific studies that have proven that the seeds of autoimmune illness are sown early in life. "The immune system can carry out the belief that on some level the body is unacceptable or unlovable and therefore attacks itself/the body. Characteristics of abortion survivors are often those who are "over-achievers, always on the go to alleviate their own self-negation, or under-achievers, certain they will not make the cut". They are the least likely of people to ask for support/help. They tend to be extremely independent. "Annihilation ideation is one of the strongest threats anyone could ever experience. It is like being hunted by a murderer or stalked by a psychopath. The primitive brain is forced into constant alert.

Panic or complete collapse is often present in a regression. Those who have experienced annihilation ideation carry a deep rooted despair about a life coupled with a fighting spirit that is undaunted by any obstacle." This perfectly described who I 'was'.

I realized by this time that the confirmation I thought I needed really no longer mattered because I had gained a greater strength in trusting what the Lord had shown me despite the fearful thoughts, comments, or worries. I was content (for a while) with this explanation. However, it was just another confirmation that GOD IS FAITHFUL AND HE WILL ALWAYS DELIVER US! The truth always leads us if we allow it.

My logical brain made it easier to believe what my heart was trying to show me. My heart has physically beaten so loudly for the past 4 years since my awareness of my prenatal life; it often kept me distracted and frustrated because that's all I could feel. Through a lot of prayer and discernment I have finally realized that God has been trying to show me to listen to my heart and not my head.

In January 2012, my family went on a ski trip and there I took a few days to complete my book. It felt good to be done but there was something that kept telling me I was not finished. Later that day I began to have headaches, each night I would wake more often with my jaws clenched. Over the next 6 weeks my headaches intensified and woke me nightly. I decided to see Margo for a physical therapy treatment and as she was doing some cranial work on me the pain intensified and she asked me, "do you think this has anything to do with working on your book lately?". The tears just started to roll down my face. I felt a lot of strong emotions and it occurred to me that my headaches started the day I finished my book. I felt relief after the treatment and the headache was gone. However, I knew I had to get my book back out and figure out what needed to be done to complete it. I continued to pray for answers, journal, and felt in my heart that I had not spoken the truth that I experienced. I tried to avoid it, but about a week later the intense headaches began waking me nightly again. My days were filling with anger and frustration for unknown reasons all over again. As I began to re-write what I experienced in my prenatal regression, peace came over me, and the headaches quickly left and I began to sleep peacefully. I would like to share this last journal entry:

> *Journal Entry 2-26-12: Thank you Lord for this beautiful day. Thank you for the wisdom you are giving me for my healing. These headaches have been very intense lately. Yesterday as the headaches intensified and the nausea set in I asked myself...." What am I holding on to that is making me sick inside?" I started weeping and felt like I couldn't stop.*

Thoughts of the truth God showed me came flooding in, my symptoms (rapid heartbeat, strong urine, losing sleep, chronic UTI, stressed adrenals, fatigue) returned. I was holding on to emotional toxicity. Obviously, I was not finished with my book. This book has been a great part of my healing- an assignment God has given me to bring healing. I realize, through His grace, that my choice to hold on to toxins is making me physically ill. The anger that left when I experienced the truth of my prenatal life returned and it was not only affecting me but all those I loved around me. Even though this experience was very traumatic to me at the earliest stages of development and again as I remembered it through my prenatal regression it brought more inner peace to me than I had had my whole life. This is a great example of God's love and teaching. Logically one would think this is absurd and makes no sense. That is the beauty of God's love, the mystery of faith. Yes, it is good to have logic and reason but if we go beyond that and trust our intuition and what is in our heart we can experience the deepest healing we have ever known. The peace we feel in the midst of chaos, that is faith and by that faith we will receive this healing. It is all in God's time and season and by the choices we make.

You see it's like driving down a road to our destination. God's path is clear with much light and signs to lead us in the right direction. Then comes curves in the road, the bumps, the potholes, and darkness that causes us to get lost. These can be seen as evil forces, spiritual attacks, or the confusion of this world. It is not easy to stay on the right path and by God's grace we have many opportunities to get back on the right path, because he never leaves us and his light shines over us leading the way so we can continue on our journey. If we allow it the curves, bumps, and darkness actually make us stronger to continue our journey. We can not look back in regret, we must look forward and continue to follow the light and accept dark paths as merely a refueling, a tune up to continue on our real journey home to Heaven.

The core of my healing has been the awareness I received in my prenatal regression. It has been anger that I held even before I knew what anger was. It has affected my liver, gall bladder (where anger is stored), and my digestion all my life. There are statistics that show colon health affects 70% of our immunity. It is crucial for absorbing nutrients our bodies need to function properly as the liver and gall bladder filter, and eliminate what was not needed. This affects our adrenal gland function (like the motor in our car), which provides our energy needed to live. So by holding in these emotional toxins I was depleting the energy needed to carry out God's will. There is really no way to prove it, nor a need to, but God has clearly shown me in order to complete this assignment I must share my story. Accepting this truth brings me great peace and releases all that keeps me ill and allows me to be the person God created me to be so I can feel love versus anger and resentment. It allows me to let God's light shine through me for all to see, which is the one thing I remember praying for before I fell ill. years ago. Logic and reason tells me this truth may be difficult for others to accept and may even be hurtful which is what caused me to change my story in the first place (a curve in my path), but truth tells me that as I trust what God has shown me I will receive and pass on greater healing beyond my imagination! He reminds me in **Luke 1:45, "Blessed are you who believed that what was spoken to you by the Lord wouid be fulfilled"**.

Every time I went to a heart doctor my best explanation was that 'I felt like I was being shocked or that I had a short circuit in my heart. I felt like someone would turn off the main breaker in me that controlled my electrical system and everything would shut down and I would proceed to blackout'. Most of the doctors looked at me with confusion or like I was crazy. As I stated earlier, one of the 'best' doctors known here in Oklahoma diagnosed me with "neurocardiogenic syncope", which he described as a nerve somewhere in the body causing this to happen but they did not know why and their fix for it was an ablation(burning of the artery) or a pacemaker. It is an answer and a temporary fix for many, but God has given me strength to seek out the truth. Through my last few physical therapy treatments with Micha and Margo I have found that by accepting and speaking the truth I experienced, my heart will be healed. After researching further, I found through notes of Dr. Mines that at 4 weeks gestation "the head and tail are formed which means there is brain and spinal cord development. Neural folds fuse and heart tubes fuse at midline. This is where the optic vessels appear, nostrils appear, and the beginning of the lungs, liver, stomach, pancreas, and thyroid. The upper limb buds appear, leg buds appear, heart development increases, and the optic lens forms." As you can see this is a crucial part of development, which is happening typically before the mother even knows she is pregnant or has just become aware of her pregnancy and where many abortions take place. This is where my cells were remembering the experience and unable to re-pattern the central nervous system (the short circuits

I felt in my heart from the memory in my brain) until I accepted the truth of my experience in what God had shown me.

Keep Hope! There is always an answer and it is in His timing which is ALWAYS PERFECT! I will end this book with the perfect song The Lord gave me the day I finally finished His masterpiece. I believe it is a song He wants each and everyone who reads this to hear because it is for you.........

"The Words I Would Say" by Sidewalk Prophets

"Three in the morning and I'm still awake
so I picked up a pen and a page.
And I started writing just what I'd say
if we were face to face

I'd tell you just what you mean to me
Tell you these simple truths

Be strong in the Lord and
Never give up hope...."

ACKNOWLEDGEMENTS

I would like to express my gratitude to all who were and continue to be a part of my healing journey. To my awesome husband for choosing to love me no matter what. For all the extra time he gave me to complete this book, and especially for never doubting me and supporting me throughout my healing journey. To my parents for choosing to give me life and planting the seed of faith I would need for this journey. To all my prayer warriors- Margo Hayes, PT, my dear friend, therapist and mentor. Special thanks to Margo for the multiple emergency prayers that sustain me through my healing.

Micha Sale, PT, friend, therapist, and mentor. Micha always gave me the hope I needed when I was ready to give up. She gave me great advice the day she told me- when it doesn't make sense or seems weird, it's probably from God. This helped tremendously through my healing because I finally realized all my answers were from God, and many were not accepted by others because they were not 'typical and understood'. I am also grateful for the many prayers she spoke over me while treating me. I thank her for the many years of classes she has provided to help me become the therapist I am today.

Vada Bradshaw who started out as a patient and little did I know what a precious friend she would become. Barbara Stomprud who also began as a patient, but was a great prayer warrior who has helped me realize my gifts through her gifts of prophecy.

Kristi Weldon, PT who I met during my first job as a PT. Little did I know we would meet up again several years later, in Micha's manual therapy classes and become great friends. She has been a great source of spiritual strength for me through her own spiritual gifts of healing.

Susan and Nancy Rooker. They were my first friends I met when I moved to Oklahoma and we continue to be great friends today. We may not see each other often due to our hectic schedules but they are the type of friends I can say will be there for me always until the day our good Lord takes me home.

My family (both biological and church), and all those that were asked to pray for me that I may not have been aware of. For those who sustained me in my darkest hours and also were there to celebrate my victories. To my wonderful, obeying children for accepting our new eating habits without to much fuss☺. Their smiles and loving hugs sustained me more than they may ever know.

My dear friend Jason for texting Bible references to me when I needed them.....right away.

My sisters who made many visits to help with the kids, cooking, and life. All I can say is everyone needs a sister!!!!!

All who helped nurse me back to health so this book could be possible. My friend Joelle Volpe who kindly offered to edit my book. She has six children of her own and a very busy schedule as a navy wife and homeschool mom. I am very grateful for her time.

And last but not least, I want to thank Dr. Johnson who helped give me the final name of this book, and for his wisdom as a physician. Dr. Johnson called me the evening of my shoulder surgery to check on me and said, "you are one RESILIENT young lady!" He told me my shoulder literally fell out of the socket as he moved it while I was under sedation. He commented that basically the only thing holding it in the socket was scar tissue. His yes to what he does as a professional is much appreciated and although he may not know it, his timing in repairing my shoulder is a crucial part of my healing journey and my ability to return to my passion of helping others. I realized that night I was not "stubborn" as others had said and I had come to believe myself, but that I am Resilient. It is only by the grace of God I continued to do all I had done with my shoulder in the condition it was in. God had plans for me and others who crossed my path and His timing is always perfect! I am so grateful for the healing and rest He has given me in preparation for all that is to come.

THANK YOU AND I AM SO GRATEFUL FOR YOU ALL!!!!!!!!!!!!

BIBLIOGRAPHY

Kippley, John F. and Sheila K. The Art of Natural Family Planning, 4th edition. Couple To Couple League International, Inc., 1996.

Kulacz, Robert and Tomas E. Levy. The Roots of Disease: Connecting Dentistry and Medicine. Xlibris Co., 2002.

Mines, Stephanie. Pre and Perinatal Psychology: Removing Primary Obstacles To EarlyDevelopment, Assessment and Treatment. Teaching Manual, 2006.

Mines, Stephanie. We Are All In Shock: How Overwhelming Experiences Shatter You and What You Can Do About It. Career Press, Inc., 2003.

Warren, Rick. Daily Inspirations For The Purpose Driven Life Journal. Zondervan Corporation, 2003.

*All Bible verses were referenced from The New American Bible. World Catholic Press, 1987.

Printed in the United States
By Bookmasters